International Series on Public Policy

Series Editors
B. Guy Peters
Department of Political Science
University of Pittsburgh
Pittsburgh, PA, USA

Philippe Zittoun
Research Professor of Political Science
LET-ENTPE, University of Lyon
Lyon, France

The International Series on Public Policy - the official series of International Public Policy Association, which organizes the International Conference on Public Policy - identifies major contributions to the field of public policy, dealing with analytical and substantive policy and governance issues across a variety of academic disciplines.

A comparative and interdisciplinary venture, it examines questions of policy process and analysis, policymaking and implementation, policy instruments, policy change & reforms, politics and policy, encompassing a range of approaches, theoretical, methodological, and/or empirical.

Relevant across the various fields of political science, sociology, anthropology, geography, history, and economics, this cutting edge series welcomes contributions from academics from across disciplines and career stages, and constitutes a unique resource for public policy scholars and those teaching public policy worldwide.

All books in the series are subject to Palgrave's rigorous peer review process: https://www.palgrave.com/gb/demystifying-peer-review/792492.

Johanna Hornung

The Institutions of Programmatic Action

Policy Programs in French and German
Health Policy

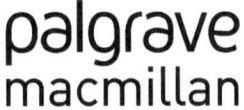

Johanna Hornung
Institute of Comparative Politics and
Public Policy
TU Braunschweig
Braunschweig, Germany

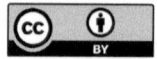

ISSN 2524-7301   ISSN 2524-731X (electronic)
International Series on Public Policy
ISBN 978-3-031-05773-1   ISBN 978-3-031-05774-8   (eBook)
https://doi.org/10.1007/978-3-031-05774-8

This Palgrave Macmillan imprint is published by the registered company Springer Nature Switzerland AG.
The registered company address is: Gewerbestrasse 11, 6330 Cham, Switzerland

To Susanne and Walter

ACKNOWLEDGMENTS

This book would not exist without the support of many people, some of whom I would like to sincerely thank explicitly. Firstly, a great thank you goes to Reimut Zohlnhöfer, my PhD supervisor, for your constructive remarks on this new theoretical perspective and the helpful feedback on how to make the most out of this dissertation project. Thank you, Georg Wenzelburger, for acting as the second evaluator of the dissertation and for giving valuable comments on an early version of this work. Thank you, Christiane Schwieren, for completing my defense committee, and for sharing the same enthusiasm for the application of psychological theories in other disciplines.

Special thanks go to Nils C. Bandelow, my mentor for many years, for extensive discussions on comparative health policy and for your outstanding support. I also thank Patrick Hassenteufel for giving me an understanding of French politics and health policy. The discussions and the work with you always inspire me and I was very happy to have the opportunity to conduct the expert interviews in France and Germany together with the two of you.

The dissertation project was embedded in a binational research project on a cross-country comparison of four national health policy trajectories—ProAcTA. Thanks go to the DFG (grant number BA 1912/3-1) and ANR (grant number ANR-17-FRAL-0008-01) for providing Nils C. Bandelow and William Genieys with funding for this project. While writing this book, I was lucky to be a member of the Comparative Politics and Public Policy team at the TU Braunschweig. I want to thank my colleagues Colette, Lisa, Derk, Ilana for being thought-provoking and supportive.

Just as much important as a scientific environment for writing a doctoral thesis are the friends who carry you through these exciting and demanding times. Thank you, Mischa, for always encouraging me in my endeavors. Thank you, Madita, Anton, Annabel, and many others—including the Rugby Welfen team in Braunschweig—for providing a distraction if needed and for holding up my work-life balance.

Finally, I am incredibly thankful for the enduring support provided by my parents, Susanne and Walter Hornung, in following the academic path. You taught me that education is our most valuable resource—thank you for always putting it first.

This book is the abridged version of a dissertation with the original title "The Institutions of Programmatic Action - Comparing and Explaining French and German Health Care Reform Programs", completed at the University of Heidelberg under the supervision of Prof. Dr. Reimut Zohlnhöfer.

The book is the result of research conducted within the project "Programmatic Action in Times of Austerity (ProAcTA)" funded by the Deutsche Forschungsgemeinschaft (DFG) (grant number BA 1912/3-1) and the Agence Nationale de la Recherche (ANR) (grant number ANR-17-FRAL-0008-01) under the direction of Prof. Dr. Nils C. Bandelow and Prof. Dr. William Genieys.

Praise for *The Institutions of Programmatic Action*

"The Programmatic Action Framework (PAF) is the newcomer in the pluralistic set of the theories of the policy process. This framework is based on the hypothesis that policy change can be driven by groups of individuals (programmatic groups), directly involved in the policy process, sharing both the definition and the solutions of policy problems and capable to behave strategically as a collective actor. This fascinating and promising hypothesis needed to be embedded into an institutional context to grasp the characteristics of programmatic groups (when and how they are formed, their ideational core and their capacity to get or not the expected policy change). This book does exactly, and convincingly, this job by focusing on those institutional conditions that shape the foundation and the space of action of programmatic groups. Thanks to a detailed and systematic comparative analysis of three decades of health policy in France and Germany, Johanna Hornung not only offers a fresh understanding of policy change in the analyzed sectors but also shows how high can be the explanatory potential of the PAF for comparative public policy."
—Prof. Dr. Giliberto Capano, *University of Bologna, Italy*

"Johanna Hornung's book is an excellent and novel application of a recently established policy process framework: the Programmatic Action Framework (PAF). The book presents empirical cross-country evidence for the PAF's idea that overlapping biographies of policy actors and resulting social identities often drive collective action. Hornung further offers an in-depth analysis of how elite recruitment, institutionalized scientific advice, and biographical commonalities among policy actors can influence long-term policy change over several decades. A central finding of this work is that programmatic groups can form in every country, but they depend more on an institutionalization of scientific advice and career recruitment than on federalist or corporatist structures that are usually viewed as moderators of policy processes."
—Prof. Dr. Tanya Heikkila, *University of Colorado Denver, USA*

"This carefully researched and argued book continues the development of the Programmatic Action Framework, an approach to policy-making built on the basis of careful examination of the situation in France where policy-making is characterized by how 'policy actors coalesce around a policy program to achieve policy change in order to advance their own authority and careers in a policy area'. The approach combines elements from public administration, elite sociology, and social psychology to help explain policy dynamics and provides many insights into how policies develop, are maintained, and change. By examining the similarities and differences between the German and French health policies, the book highlights how program coalitions and activities in each country differ in terms of socialization and elite formation – which in Germany promotes cross-program identities as lawyers or party politicians rather than purely program proponents – and in the degree of institutionalized involvement of expert advice in the policy process. This work advances knowledge of programmatic actors comparatively and, as such, moves understanding of the central concept of this promising approach to policy studies forward."

—Prof. Dr. Michael Howlett, *Simon Fraser University, Canada*

"Institutionalism meets the Programmatic Action Framework. Johanna Hornung's in-depth comparative study is a must-read to understand under which conditions the interplay between institutions and programmatic actors changes French and German health policies from 1990 to 2020. Hornung shows that policy change is irrevocably linked to the programmatic group, framed by two specific institutions—the recruitment processes and career paths of administrative actors."

—Prof. Dr. Sabine Saurugger, *SciencesPo Grenoble, France*

CONTENTS

Contents

Abbreviations

ACF	Advocacy Coalition Framework
AOK	Allgemeine Ortskrankenkasse (Local Sickness Fund)
AOK-BV	AOK-Bundesverband (Federal Association of Local Sickness Funds)
AMNOG	Arzneimittelmarktneuordnungsgesetz (Pharmaceutical Market Restructuring Act)
ANSM	Agence Nationale de Sécurité du Médicament et des Produits de Santé (National Agency of Medicine and Health Products Safety)
ARS	Agences Régionales de Santé (Regional Health Agencies)
BAS	Bundesamt für Soziale Sicherung (Federal Office for Social Security); formerly Bundesversicherungsamt (Federal Insurance Office)
CADES	Caisse d'Amortissement de la Dette Sociale (Social Debt Amortisation Fund)
CDU	Christlich Demokratische Union Deutschlands (Christian Democratic Union, party in Germany)
CHT	Communautés Hospitalières Territoriales (Territorial Hospital Communities)
CNAM	Caisse Nationale de l'Assurance Maladie (National Health Insurance Fund)
CNAMTS	Caisse Nationale d'Assurance Maladie des Travailleurs Salariés (National Sickness Fund for Employed)
CNAVTS	Caisse Nationale d'Assurance-vieillesse des Travailleurs Salaries (National Old-Age Insurance Fund for Salaried Employees)
CNS	Conférence Nationale de Santé (National Health Conference)
CPTS	Communautés Professionnelles Territoriales de Santé (Territorial Professional Health Communities)

CSU	Christlich-Soziale Union (Christian Social Union, party in Germany)
DGOS	Direction Générale de l'Offre de Soins (General Directorate of Health Care Supplies)
DGS	Direction Générale de Santé (General Directorate of Health)
DKG	Deutsche Krankenhausgesellschaft (German Hospital Association)
DL	Démocratie Libérale (Liberal Democracy, party in France)
DMP	Disease Management Program
DNA	Discourse Network Analyzer
DREES	Direction de la Recherche, des Études, de l'Évaluation et des Statistiques (Research, Studies, Evaluation and Statistics Branch
DRG	Diagnosis-related Groups (Hospital remuneration system based on flat rates per case)
DSS	Direction de la Sécurité Sociale (Division of Social Security)
DVG	Digitale-Versorgung-Gesetz (Digital Care Act)
ENA	École Nationale d'Administration (National School of Administration)
EU	European Union
FDP	Freie Demokratische Partei (Liberal Democratic Party, in Germany)
FO	Force Ouvrière (Workers' Force, union in France)
G-BA	Gemeinsamer Bundesausschuss (Federal Joint Committee)
GHT	Groupements Hospitaliers de Territoire (Regional Hospital Groups)
GKV-WSG	GKV-Wettbewerbsstärkungsgesetz (Act to Strengthen Competition in the SHI)
GKV-SV	GKV-Spitzenverband (SHI Peak Association)
GKV-VEG	GKV-Versichertenentlastungsgesetz (Act to Relieve the Burden on Insured Persons in SHI)
GMG	GKV-Modernisierungsgesetz (SHI Modernization Act)
GRG	Gesundheitsreformgesetz (Health Care Reform Act)
GSG	Gesundheitsstrukturgesetz (Health Care Structure Act)
HAS	Haute Autorité de Santé (National Health Authority)
HCAAM	Haut Conseil pour l'Avenir de l'Assurance Maladie (High Council for the Future of Health Insurance)
HPST	Loi Hôpital, Patients, Santé, Territoires (Hospital, Patients, Health Territories Act)
IRDES	Institut de Recherche et Documentation en Économie de la Santé (Institute for Research and Information in Health Economics)
IQWIG	Institut für Qualität und Wirtschaftlichkeit im Gesundheitswesen (Institute for Quality and Efficiency in Health Care)

KBV	Kassenärztliche Bundesvereinigung (Federal Association of Sickness Fund Physicians)
LMSS	Loi de Modernisation de notre Système de Santé (Health System Modernisation Act)
LREM	La République En Marche (The Republic on the Move, party in France)
MSF	Multiple Streams Framework
NA	National Assembly (in France)
NPF	Narrative Policy Framework
ONDAM	Objectif National des Dépenses d'Assurance Maladie (National Objective of Sickness Fund Expenditures)
PAF	Programmatic Action Framework
PFT	Policy Feedback Theory
PLFSS	Projet de Loi de Financement de la Sécurité Sociale (Financing Laws of the Social Security
PpSG	Pflegepersonalstärkungsgesetz (Act to Strengthen the Nursing Staff)
PS	Parti Socialiste (Socialist Party, in France)
ROSP	Rémunération sur Objectifs de Santé Publique (Remuneration for General Practitioners Based on Public Health Objectives)
RPR	Rassemblement pour la République (Rally for the Republic, party in France)
RSA	Risikostrukturausgleich (risk structure compensation)
SCT	Self-Categorization Theory
SHI	Statutory Health Insurance
SIA	Social Identity Approach; Combination of SCT and SIT
SIPP	Social Identities in the Policy Process
SIT	Social Identity Theory
SPD	Sozialdemokratische Partei Deutschland (Social Democratic Party in Germany)
SVR-G	Sachverständigenrat zur Begutachtung der Entwicklung im Gesundheitswesen (Council of Experts on the Assessment of Developments in the Health Care System)
UDF	Union pour la Démocratie Française (Union for the French Democracy, party in France)
UK	United Kingdom
UMP	Union pour la Majorité Présidentielle (Union for the Presidential Majority, party in France)
UNCAM	Union Nationale des Caisses d'Assurance Maladie (National Union of Health Insurance Funds)
US	United States
WIdO	Wissenschaftliches Institut der AOK (Scientific Institute of Local Sickness Funds)

LIST OF FIGURES

LIST OF TABLES

List of Tables

CHAPTER 1

Introduction

In the 1970s' Chile, neoliberal reform ideas entered economic policy under Augusto Pinochet, who took power in the then Marxist-dominated country in 1973. The roots of this change are traced back to the so-called Chicago Boys, who—although born in Chile—were educated at the University of Chicago as part of a cooperation with the Universidad Catolica and later spread the monetarist ideas in key positions in academia, business, and politics (Brender, 2010; Kogut & Macpherson, 2008). While there is a consensus that they can be described as technocrats who brought neoliberal thinking into Chilean government and society, some even see them as "revolutionary vanguard" (Clark, 2017). Importantly, however, both members and non-members of the group refer to them as the "Chicago Boys" and irrevocably associate them with a set of policy ideas. As such, they exemplify the impact that a shared biographical connection, based on shared education, for example, can have on long-term cooperation and change in policy.

Biographical ties and a resulting sense of belonging associated with policy ideas thus have the potential to influence long-term interactions between individuals. The Programmatic Action Framework (PAF) is a comparatively recent perspective that integrates this idea into policy process research (Bandelow et al., 2021; Hassenteufel & Genieys, 2021). By systematically incorporating elements from public administration, elite sociology, and social psychology (particularly the role of social identities),

J. Hornung, *The Institutions of Programmatic Action*,
International Series on Public Policy,
https://doi.org/10.1007/978-3-031-05774-8_1

the PAF adds a complementary lens to explain policy change and stability. With regard to the former, the PAF integrates the assumption that the actors close to the bureaucratic state apparatus exert a direct influence on policy formulation. The sociology of elites sees the trajectories of policy actors as roots for their behavior, which is taken up in the PAF by looking at shared biographies as a source of cooperation between policy actors. Finally, the Social Identities in the Policy Process (SIPP) perspective (Hornung et al., 2019) provides an explanation for the long-term stability of social groups based on distinct social identities. These can include biographical/demographic identities, but—in the long run—also programmatic identities, which specifically refer to groups that form around a policy program. The observation that so-called programmatic groups push their policy programs until they achieve policy change is called programmatic action and gives the framework its name.

Research has noted that the shape of programmatic groups may vary depending on the political institutions in which they form (Hassenteufel et al., 2010), but has so far not addressed how these institutions influence the occurrence of programmatic action. However, to make the theoretical perspective a valuable addition to comparative public policy, it is indispensable to reflect on the institutional conditions necessary for programmatic action to be observed. This gap will be filled by this study by answering the question: *Under which institutional conditions programmatic action does occur in the first place and how do political institutions contribute to the success or failure of programmatic groups?* Given that the PAF has evolved from the programmatic approach, which was originally developed against the background of French policy-making and the specificities of the French political system, one might think that the PAF represents a unique account of French policy processes. However, PAF applications to other political systems with different institutional settings in terms of federalism, corporatism, and the structure of policy sectors show that the PAF actually demonstrates some traveling capacity across countries and policy fields (Davidian, 2021; Duque, 2021; Hornung & Bandelow, 2020). The present study complements PAF research with a systematic analysis of the institutional preconditions necessary for programmatic action to come about. It thus answers the question of the institutional conditions under which programmatic action takes place—an endeavor that has not yet been explicitly considered in previous research.

To this end, a systematic analysis of instances of programmatic action in two institutionally different states is conducted: France and Germany. This selection is based—in addition to the institutionally different conditions—on the premise that programmatic action has already been observed in these countries (Genieys & Hassenteufel, 2015; Hornung & Bandelow, 2020). The policy area on which the analysis focuses is that of health policy, partly because health policy is particularly suited to outlining institutional conditions of federalism and corporatism that are less visible in other policy areas.

1.1   Theoretical and Empirical Puzzle

Although formally established in 2018, the PAF's ideational history dates back to the earliest studies of programmatic actors within the programmatic approach. Focusing on the evolution of French health policy since the 1980s, Genieys and Hassenteufel (2015) conducted a seminal study of what he called the emergence of a new welfare elite. He characterized this elite in terms of joint training at the École Nationale d'Administration (ENA) (National School of Administration) and mutual cooperation when these elite actors later occupied key positions in the French government. The welfare elite vigorously defended the health care sector against the austerity measures proposed by the "austerians", which followed exactly the strategy exemplified by Ronald Reagan and Margaret Thatcher to dismantle the welfare state (Jensen et al., 2019). By protecting the social policy sector from the effects of these measures, the actors of the welfare elite were appropriately called the "new custodians of state" (Genieys, 2010). Protecting the state in this context means not only maintaining social spending to ensure financial strength, but also maintaining regulatory powers and authority in the social security sector (Genieys & Joana, 2017, p. 332). This relates to what has been explained in the discussion of the dismantling of the welfare state as the size of the public sector and administration, paradoxically a strong state as a result of neoliberal reforms (Gamble, 1994).

The neoliberal turn with which this introductory chapter opened was thus not only visible in Chilean economic policy under the influence of the Chicago Boys. At least since the 1970s or 1980s, welfare state policies in industrialized countries have entered an era of austerity (Finseraas & Vernby, 2011; Pierson, 2002). This is visible through the increasing use of cost-containment measures (Bonoli & Natali, 2012, p. 6), thus underpinning the argument of a neoliberal direction in which social policy has been moving since then (Rynei, 2009). In the Anglo-Saxon countries of the

United States (US) and the United Kingdom (UK), retrenchment and austerity reforms were adopted under Thatcher and Reagan, respectively, with the goal of dismantling the welfare state, but they largely did not produce the desired results (Pierson, 1994; Starke, 2006, p. 105).

The conflict between custodians and austerians is very specific to the French case and an ideal-typical pattern that rooted primarily in the analysis of biographical trajectories. Depending on the positions the actors took in the social security or financing sector, they can be assigned to one of the two sides of the conflict. The analysis thus followed a sociological research design of elite research. Adapting this lens to policy research and countries other than France therefore requires a generalization of the conflict presented and a modification of the actor concept. As the programmatic approach was modified in light of the emerging PAF, the term elite was later dropped in favor of the framework-related terms programmatic actor (individual actor) or programmatic group (collective actor). This not only facilitates the delineation of actors by circumventing the need to define what comprises an "elite", but also ensures transferability to other political and education systems, where elite thinking is less inherent.

To briefly clarify the roots of the "programmatic" term: The original perspective on "custodians" versus "austerians" was associated with the idea that the two sides were advancing different policy programs—long-term strategies and visions in shaping the health care sector—one pursuing the path of neoliberal austerity and the other that of social protection. The programmatic approach assumed competition between elite actors who formulate their views on the sector through policy programs and use their intellectual and power resources to implement them (Genieys & Hassenteufel, 2015, p. 281f). At least in health policy, reform paths seemed to follow a coherent policy program of a group of programmatic actors who used their resources to implement their ideas and compete against the so-called austerians in the struggle for authority.

Although the genesis of the PAF starts from a very specific institutional setting of French policy-making, with a powerful bureaucracy and an executive elevated by the ENA, programmatic action also occurred in German health policy, characterized by completely different institutional characteristics of both the political and the health care system. Looking at the policy processes in German health policy since the 1980s, there are interconnected policies that presumably follow a common coherent thread—a policy program—that cannot be explained by existing theoretical perspectives in policy process research (Hornung & Bandelow, 2020).

Between the early 1990s and 2011, a programmatic group around the program "Competition in a Solidaristic Framework" (Knieps, 2017, p. 12) shaped German health policy (Hornung & Bandelow, 2020). The current version of the PAF has overcome the divide between "custodians" and "austerians" visible in France and adds to policy process research in general the explanation of programmatic action for policy change. The applicability of the PAF in policy process research has since been tested in several studies. However, although existing research demonstrates the applicability of the PAF in different institutional contexts, it is still under-theorized and insufficiently explored which institutional predispositions actually enable or hinder programmatic action. It is this theoretical and empirical puzzle this study ties in with.

As a consequence of the above puzzle, the guiding research question to be answered in this contribution arises systematically from the theoretical under-specification of the PAF in terms of the institutional opportunities and constraints of programmatic action and the empirical puzzle of why the PAF has developed the same explanatory power in terms of observed policy processes and policy outputs in the most diverse institutional settings of France and Germany. The overarching research question is therefore:

> *Under what institutional conditions does programmatic action take place? In other words: Under what institutional conditions do programmatic groups form on the basis of shared biographies and influence the policy process from policy formulation to policy adoption with their pursued policy program?*

Specifically, and in concretization of this research question, it is also the central aim of this study to investigate which circumstances enable or hinder programmatic action, from programmatic group formation to programmatic success. To what extent do political institutions contribute to the success and failure of programmatic groups? The argument to be defended is that programmatic groups can form in any country, regardless of structural, institutional, and political embeddedness, but that certain institutions facilitate and hinder the formation and success of programmatic groups and policy programs. The empirical analysis will identify generalizable institutional conditions that are necessary for the emergence of programmatic action. The innovative contribution to policy process research consists above all in the fact that the institutions that are relevant for programmatic action are not the same as those usually considered in the fields of comparative politics and policy process research.

Answering the research question posed provides insights into processes of policy-making in contemporary France and Germany. It must be emphasized, however, that while observing parallel programmatic action in French and German health policy over a period of time may support the usefulness of the PAF, it does not equate to universal applicability of the PAF in every context. It merely supports the claim that PAF offers explanatory power in cases where other policy process frameworks tend to overlook important explanatory aspects, namely biographical trajectories and social identities connected to policy programs. This does not preclude, but in fact supports, the claim that PAF may well fail in other cases, where other theoretical perspectives fit much better.

1.2   Methodology

To gain insights into the processes of policy-making and the institutions that drive programmatic action, it is necessary to conduct an in-depth analysis of these processes. Since the research questions do not aim at examining average effects of variables on outcomes, but take a process perspective on the institutions of programmatic action and thus require fundamental insights into the policy process, a qualitative research design suggests itself. There is a standardized procedure for a study of programmatic action that includes six steps divided into three main tasks (see Fig. 1.1). These consist of a positional and sociological analysis of programmatic actors, an analysis of the links between programmatic actors and a policy program, and an analysis of the power of the programmatic group in terms of its resources and impact in the overall policy process (Hassenteufel & Genieys, 2021).

Institutions can be relevant at any level of this research protocol. They indicate the key positions that actors must occupy and influence the trajectories that policy actors reveal, they can be an expression of policy programs and a frame for programmatic actors to promote their policy program within. They can be critical in the allocation of resources to programmatic actors and influence the implementation of the policy program. Consequently, each of the three steps is carried out for the cases of programmatic action studied in order to be able to uncover the institutional effects on the whole process of programmatic action. To this end, the empirical analysis draws on several data sources. Official legislative texts, documents of the legislative process, and public reports and newspaper articles are used to identify programs. In addition, biographical files and

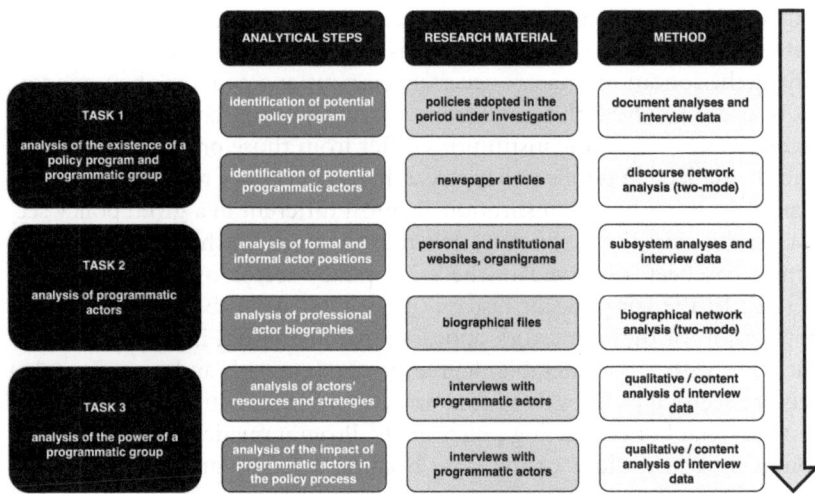

Fig. 1.1 Research protocol of programmatic action in policy process research. Source: Own visualization, slightly modified on the basis of Hassenteufel and Genieys (2021, p. 34)

information from government or analytical documents are used to analyze actors. Finally, interviews are used to obtain information about the entire process of programmatic action; these also include insider information and regular (informal) exchanges with actors in the health system. In particular, the expert interviews with key actors make it possible to gain a conclusive impression of the precise institutional opportunities and constraints they faced during their time as programmatic actors. It is therefore possible to augment valid information with interviews with actors who were directly involved in the policy-making process to illustrate the roots and trajectory of reforms under different institutional conditions. The multiple use of data from documents, publications, and expert interviews ensures validity and reliability by cross-checking information obtained through one method with information extracted from the other.

However, before proceeding with the analysis, it is necessary to present a reasoned case selection that allows the subsequent findings to be placed in the adequate context of generalization. To this end, the study is comparative in nature and follows a case selection based on the method of agreement dating back to Mill (1848). This method suggests that to explain the same phenomenon (programmatic action), a selection of cases with largely varying conditions (in this case institutional) allows for identifying the conditions that are necessary circumstances for the phenomenon.

In order to reveal the institutions relevant to programmatic action and to emphasize that these institutions differ from those prominently known and thematized in public policy research, it is necessary to select for empirical study cases that are institutionally most different in a given policy sector. At the same time, however, they must be cases in which programmatic action has been observed in the same policy sector over a similar time period. In the fairly recent history of the PAF, it has been noted that an application of the framework appears most promising in sectors close to the state with a considerable degree of state control, and in sectors that require sectoral policies to address structural, organizational challenges of fundamental but conflicting policy goals. Programmatic groups are rather found in sectors close to the state because a programmatic group must involve bureaucrats and, where appropriate, members of indirect public administration (self-governance) to bring together diverse resources and positions that enable coherent and consistent implementation of the policy program. Sectors close to the state are those in which the state acts not only as a regulator but also as a provider of services. Striking examples are health policy, education policy, and transportation policy (Mayntz & Scharpf, 1995). In these fields, a policy program developed by actors within the state administration and other sectoral actors is more likely to prevail than in policy areas where market-based governance is more present. PAF analyses focusing on health policy have been conducted in the different national settings of Spain, the UK, the US, France, and Germany (Hassenteufel et al., 2010; Hornung & Bandelow, 2020).

Taking these examples as a starting point and sticking to the policy sector of health policy, this analysis will take a closer look at two cases: The French and German political systems are characterized by a great divergence with regard to their institutions. On both the executive-parties dimension and the federal-unitary dimension of Lijphart's classification of types of democracy, France and Germany each occupy the other half of the scale, placing them in the opposite quadrants of the coordinate system for both dimensions (Lijphart, 2012, pp. 244-245). France and Germany thus differ in many respects: France is characterized by a pluralistic interest group system, centralized decision-making processes, a government with a strong executive in a semi-presidential system, and a majoritarian electoral system. Germany is a parliamentary democracy with a special role for subnational states ("Länder") through the second legislative body of the Bundesrat, a tradition of strong corporatist settings, and a proportional representation electoral system. In particular, the opportunity structures for policy actors inherent in federalism, corporatism, and the adjunct number of veto players are most different and therefore provide policy actors with different opportunities to pursue strategies in policy-making. The selection of France and Germany as case studies therefore follows the call of public policy scholars to select cases that say something about the link between systems and phenomena and to use the cases to systematically reveal these connections (van der Heijden, 2014, p. 36).

As regards the period of analysis, there are clear analyses of the French programmatic elite in health policy that emerged in the 1980s and secured its influence on policy-making at least until the mid-2000s (Genieys & Hassenteufel, 2015). The health care reform under Nicolas Sarkozy, entitled the Hospital, Patients, Health, and Territories Act (Loi Hôpital, Patients, Santé et Territoires; HPST), was also part of this ongoing success of a welfare elite toward a strengthened state in times of austerity (Simonet, 2018, p. 3). It is this welfare elite that will be the focus of later empirical analysis in order to understand what institutional conditions enabled its continued success. Continued because even in the current situation of the Corona crisis, the programmatic group appears to continue to have influence (Hassenteufel, 2020). The period of analysis in France spans from 1990 to 2020, a total of 30 years.

In Germany, the duration of the programmatic group was somewhat shorter, although it is debatable whether reforms in the 2010s can still be counted under the policy program label. The Pharmaceutical Market Restructuring Act (Arzneimittelmarktneuordnungsgesetz, AMNOG) appears to be the most recent health care reform that clearly falls under the program of introducing competition into the health care system with the goal of increasing cost efficiency and solidarity (Dingermann, 2013; Herr, 2013). Although the vision of competition seemed unbroken in 2014 (Manzei et al., 2014), the legislative period under health minister Hermann Gröhe 2013–2017 did not continue this line (Bandelow et al., 2019, p. 463). For this reason, the period between 1990 and 2011 is analyzed for the German case. However, in order to determine, in the true sense, the institutional factors that favor programmatic action, it is also necessary to examine a case in which programmatic action did not occur. In this case, too, the institutional circumstances should lead to the expected result. Therefore, the period after programmatic action in Germany, from

2011 onward, is also included in the analysis. The fact that the period of analysis from 2010 onward in the aftermath of the financial crisis shows a persistence of the programmatic group in France and an end to the programmatic group in Germany makes it all the more possible to clarify the institutional conditions of programmatic action.

In order to analyze the factors of success, it is necessary to define what a successful programmatic group and policy program are. Success is multidimensional and can refer to the realm of process, program, and politics (McConnell, 2010). Specifically, program and political success are relevant to PAF, but in a different understanding than in existing research. Since programmatic actors are not elected and thus cannot achieve political in terms of electoral success, their success is defined by having more authority and resources in the sector. Thus, a programmatic group is successful if its members move up the career ladder, hold key positions in the sector for a long time, and have resources (both financial and regulatory) to influence their policy sector. Indicators of financial and regulatory resources would be increased budgetary importance to their policy sector (e.g., increased spending) and an increased policy authority for health care decision-making.

The success of a policy program in terms of the PAF is unrelated to a normative outcome, that is, an assessment of whether the adoption and implementation of a policy has led to the desired result, at least insofar as it does not affect the overall goals of the policy program. To give an example, if the vision of the policy program is greater interlocking of care across sectors, and one reform step is the establishment of medical care centers overseen by multiple institutions to coordinate care across sectors, it is not of interest to the programmatic group promoting the policy program whether these medical care centers actually improve care in a normative sense by, for example, ensuring access to specialists or improving quality of medical interventions. As long as the overall goal of a closer sector integration, which is the vision of the policy program, is achieved, policy outcomes and evaluations such as good or bad policy are of secondary, not primary, interest. Policy program success is defined here as the adoption of a policy program and its persistence, which is completely independent of normative effects but depends solely on the interests of the programmatic actors who profit from its implementation (Wenzelburger & Zohlnhöfer, 2015, p. 19).

Revealing the factors of success of programmatic groups and policy programs that are embedded in the institutions that enable or hinder programmatic action is the central research interest of this study. However, while the success of policy programs and programmatic actors is easier to determine with an outside perspective, understanding the role of institutions is only possible by gaining a detailed picture of the policy process through inside information. Therefore, expert interviews with programmatic actors identified in the previous two analytical steps were chosen as the research material and method for this final analytical task. The interviews also subsequently allow validation of the previously generated results on the policy program and programmatic actors.

1.3 OUTLINE

Taken these considerations together, it is worth recapitulating what this book does and does not aim to do. Starting from the observation that programmatic action occurred in the health care systems of France and Germany despite their most different institutional designs, the main argument to be advanced in the following chapters is that there are institutional predispositions in each nation that allow for the formation of programmatic groups and the resulting promotion and implementation of their policy program over several years. While there is already evidence of programmatic action in France and Germany during the period of observation, it has not yet been systematically analyzed what institutional factors enabled programmatic action. This is particularly relevant given that the political institutions of federalism, corporatism, and party systems differ considerably in the two states. To what extent can the institutional preconditions be generalized on a broader level to make PAF applicable beyond the French, German, and European borders? To achieve this goal, the main contribution of this book is to conduct a detailed systematic and comparative analysis of the presence and absence of programmatic action in French and German health policy over the past 30 years, and to identify the commonalities that have enabled this programmatic action in France and Germany.

It is worth noting that the analysis of programmatic action is possible by starting from one of the two sides of the pole: programmatic actors or policy programs. Given that this book is situated in the field of policy process research, the variable of interest remains policies. Consequently, the empirical analysis begins with a systematic overview on relevant sectoral policies. It devotes its attention, firstly, to the analysis of policy programs that encompass a consistent and coherent vision for the health sector, realized in separate but few comprehensive acts, accompanied only by minor adaptive measures. Secondly, tracing this vision back to the actors and the ideational roots of its content, the analysis reveals personal connections between actors and major, comprehensive health reforms, rather than those that only entail regulations for a very specific aspect of the health care sector (e.g., hospitals) without affecting another. Network graphs visualize the biographical links between programmatic actors. The underlying data stem from systematic analyses of official documents and biographical files, as well as interviews. Thirdly and finally, these interviews with key informants and members of the programmatic groups are used to address the central research interest, to uncover the policy processes during each period of programmatic action, with a specific focus on the institutional opportunities and constraints that led to the formation of these programmatic groups and that they faced in realizing their policy program. Thirty-one qualitative in-depth interviews reveal which institutions proved conducive to programmatic action and thus relevant to the ultimate formation of programmatic groups, their policy programs, and the success of both.

Although the health policy sector under investigation is related to the welfare state, the study conducted does not directly aim to explain welfare state retrenchment or expansion. As such, it is not designed to provide explanations for why a specific content of reforms was chosen, apart from question of the extent to which the content can be considered as an explanatory factor for the success of the policy program. Rather, the analysis sheds light on the opportunities and constraints that programmatic groups faced when promoting their policy program, both regarding the institutionally pertinent factors for programmatic group formation and programmatic groups' as well as programs' success, and regarding the group-specific and program-specific characteristics that facilitated that success.

Overall, this book is divided into four parts, of which this introduction is the first. The second part is devoted to theory. This first covers the theoretical foundations of the PAF laid in Chap. 2 ("Programmatic Action and Policy Processes"), including the debates to which it contributes and a delineation of the PAF from existing perspectives. Following this preliminary work, Chap. 3 ("Political Institutions and Public Policy") links the PAF to existing institutional perspectives and derives hypotheses about the potential influence of institutions on programmatic action. Hence, this chapter is particularly designed to highlight the institutional circumstances that are typically assumed to influence policy-making and potentially explain the occurrence of programmatic action in the two countries. Based on the interim conclusion on the influence of institutions, the empirical part (part III) contains a detailed analysis of programmatic action in France and Germany (Chaps. 5 and 6), after having provided an overview of the institutional settings of health policy in the two countries (Chap. 4). The last part consists of two concluding chapters: The first summarizes the results of the empirical analysis with respect to programmatic action in France and Germany with a view on the institutions necessary for programmatic action (Chap. 7). The second (Chap. 8) answers the overarching research question which commonalities in most different political systems are drivers of programmatic action and thus facilitate or hinder the emergence and success of programmatic groups and policy programs. It also addresses the challenge of institutional change to programmatic action before emphasizing the limitations and directions for future PAF research that result from the study.

REFERENCES

Bandelow, N. C., Hartmann, A., & Hornung, J. (2019). Selbstbeschränkte Gesundheitspolitik im Vorfeld neuer Punktuierungen. In R. Zohlnhöfer & T. Saalfeld (Eds.), *Zwischen Stillstand, Politikwandel und Krisenmanagement: Eine Bilanz der Regierung Merkel 2013-2017* (pp. 445–467). Springer Fachmedien Wiesbaden.

Bandelow, N. C., Hornung, J., & Smyrl, M. (2021). Theoretical Foundations of the Programmatic Action Framework (PAF). *European Policy Analysis, 7*(1), 14–27. https://doi.org/10.1002/epa2.1083

Bonoli, G., & Natali, D. (2012). The Politics of the 'New' Welfare States. In G. Bonoli & D. Natali (Eds.), *The Politics of the New Welfare State* (pp. 3–19). Oxford University Press.

Brender, V. (2010). Economic Transformations in Chile: The Formation of the Chicago Boys. *The American Economist, 55*(1), 111–122. https://doi.org/10.1177/056943451005500112

Clark, T. D. (2017). Rethinking Chile's 'Chicago Boys': Neoliberal Technocrats or Revolutionary Vanguard? *Third World Quarterly, 38*(6), 1350–1365. https://doi.org/10.1080/01436597.2016.1268906

Davidian, A. (2021). Health Reform in Brazil: The Sanitaristas as Programmatic Actors. *European Policy Analysis, 7*(1), 64–95.

Dingermann, T. (2013). Das Arzneimittelmarktneuordnungsgesetz (AMNOG) und seine Folgen. *Der Internist, 54*(6), 769–774. https://doi.org/10.1007/s00108-013-3247-2

Duque, J. F. (2021). Who Embodies the Evaluative State? Programmatic Elites in the Chilean and the Colombian Policies of Quality Assurance in Higher Education. *European Policy Analysis, 7*(1), 48–63.

Finseraas, H., & Vernby, K. (2011). What Parties Are and What Parties Do: Partisanship and Welfare State Reform in an Era of Austerity. *Socio-Economic Review, 9*(4), 613–638. https://doi.org/10.1093/ser/mwr003

Gamble, A. (1994). *The Free Economy and the Strong State. The Politics of Thatcherism*. Palgrave Macmillan.

Genieys, W. (2010). *The New Custodians of the State: Programmatic Elites in French Society*. Transaction Publishers.

Genieys, W., & Hassenteufel, P. (2015). The Shaping of New State Elites: Healthcare Policymaking in France Since 1981. *Comparative Politics, 47*(3), 280–295. Retrieved from http://www.jstor.org/stable/43664147

Genieys, W., & Joana, J. (2017). The Custodians of State Policies Dealing With the Financial Crisis: A Comparison Between France and the US. *International Relations and Diplomacy, 5*(5), 322–341.

Hassenteufel, P. (2020). Handling the COVID-19 Crisis in France: Politicization and Policy Changes in a Centralized State-led Health System. *European Policy Analysis, 6*(2), 1.

Hassenteufel, P., & Genieys, W. (2021). The Programmatic Action Framework: An Empirical Assessment. *European Policy Analysis, 7*(1), 28–47. https://doi.org/10.1002/epa2.1088

Hassenteufel, P., Smyrl, M., Genieys, W., & Moreno-Fuentes, F. J. (2010). Programmatic Actors and the Transformation of European Health Care States. *Journal of Health Politics, Policy and Law, 35*(4), 517–538. https://doi.org/10.1215/03616878-2010-015

Herr, A. (2013). Wettbewerb und Rationalisierung im deutschen Arzneimittel markt: Ein Überblick. *List Forum für Wirtschafts- und Finanzpolitik, 39*(2), 163–181. https://doi.org/10.1007/BF03373047

Hornung, J., & Bandelow, N. C. (2020). The Programmatic Elite in German Health Policy: Collective Action and Sectoral History. *Public Policy and Administration, 35*(3), 247–265. https://doi.org/10.1177/0952076718798887

Hornung, J., Bandelow, N. C., & Vogeler, C. S. (2019). Social Identities in the Policy Process. *Policy Sciences, 52*(2), 211–231. https://doi.org/10.1007/s11077-018-9340-6

Jensen, C., Wenzelburger, G., & Zohlnhöfer, R. (2019). Dismantling the Welfare State? After Twenty-five Years: What Have We Learned and What Should We

Learn? *Journal of European Social Policy, 29*(5), 681–691. https://doi.org/10.1177/0958928719877363

Knieps, F. (2017). *Gesundheitspolitik: Akteure, Aufgaben, Lösungen.* MWV Medizinisch Wissenschaftliche Verlagsgesellschaft mbH & Company KG.

Kogut, B., & Macpherson, J. M. (2008). The Decision to Privatize: Economists and the Construction of Ideas and Policies. In B. A. Simmons, F. Dobbin, & G. Garrett (Eds.), *The Global Diffusion of Markets and Democracy* (pp. 104–140). Cambridge University Press.

Lijphart, A. (2012). *Patterns of Democracy: Government Forms and Performance in Thirty-Six Countries* (2nd ed.). Yale University Press.

Manzei, A., Schnabel, M., & Schmiede, R. (2014). Embedded Competition – Oder wie kann man die Auswirkungen wettbewerblicher Regulierung im Gesundheitswesen messen? In A. Manzei & R. Schmiede (Eds.), *20 Jahre Wettbewerb im Gesundheitswesen: Theoretische und empirische Analysen zur Ökonomisierung von Medizin und Pflege* (pp. 11–31). Springer Fachmedien Wiesbaden.

Mayntz, R., & Scharpf, F. W. (Eds.). (1995). *Gesellschaftliche Selbstregelung und politische Steuerung* (Vol. 23). Campus.

McConnell, A. (2010). Policy Success, Policy Failure and Grey Areas In-Between. *Journal of Public Policy, 30*(3), 345–362. https://doi.org/10.1017/S0143814X10000152

Mill, J. S. (1848). *A System of Logic, Ratiocinative and Inductive; Being A Connected View of the Principles of Evidence and the Methods of Scientific Investigation.* Harper & Brothers.

Pierson, P. (1994). *Dismantling the Welfare State?: Reagan, Thatcher, and the Politics of Retrenchment.* Cambridge University Press.

Pierson, P. (2002). Coping with Permanent Austerity: Welfare State Restructuring in Affluent Democracies. *Revue Française de Sociologie, 43*(2), 369–406. https://doi.org/10.2307/3322510

Ryner, M. (2009). Neoliberal European Governance and the Politics of Welfare State Retrenchment: A Critique of the New Malthusians. In B. van Apeldoorn, J. Drahokoupil, & L. Horn (Eds.), *Contradictions and Limits of Neoliberal European Governance: From Lisbon to Lisbon* (pp. 44–63). Palgrave Macmillan UK.

Simonet, D. (2018). Vertical Alignment, Elite Power, and the Democratic Recess in the French Health Care System. *International Journal of Public Administration, 41*(13), 1095–1106. https://doi.org/10.1080/01900692.2017.1318918

Starke, P. (2006). The Politics of Welfare State Retrenchment: A Literature Review. *Social Policy & Administration, 40*(1), 104–120. https://doi.org/10.1111/j.1467-9515.2006.00479.x

van der Heijden, J. (2014). Selecting Cases and Inferential Types in Comparative Public Policy Research. In I. Engeli & C. R. Allison (Eds.), *Comparative Policy Studies: Conceptual and Methodological Challenges* (pp. 35–56). Palgrave Macmillan UK.

Wenzelburger, G., & Zohlnhöfer, R. (2015). Konzepte und Begriffe in der Vergleichenden Policy-Forschung. In G. Wenzelburger & R. Zohlnhöfer (Eds.), *Handbuch Poilcy-Forschung* (pp. 15–32). Springer VS.

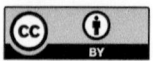

CHAPTER 2

Programmatic Action and Policy Processes

The Programmatic Action Framework (PAF) is a theoretical lens on policy processes developed at the intersection of policy process research, public administration, elite sociology, and social psychology. This chapter is particularly devoted to outlining the foundations of the PAF and putting them in context with other existing theories of the policy process. There are two main bases of PAF assumptions: Firstly, the role of bureaucracy in areas close to the state in formulating policy and the related desire for increased authority gained through advancement in individual careers. Secondly, social psychological perspectives on social identities of groups formed on the basis of shared characteristics are adopted by the PAF to outline the role of shared biographies and resulting policy programs, which are identity-forming, in policy processes and policy change. The particular focus of this study is on the institutional conditions under which such actors form programmatic groups and use their policy programs to shape the policy process over time.

In policy process research, the perspective on shared biographies and the associated promotion of policies has only marginally found its way into recent research. To be sure, there are theoretical perspectives that shed light on the question of why policy actors cooperate in policy processes. Rational choice theorists argue that collective action is a result of strategic consideration, which individual behavior generates—or promises to generate—the maximum benefit for a policy actor. In the original

© The Author(s) 2022   17
J. Hornung, *The Institutions of Programmatic Action*,
International Series on Public Policy,
https://doi.org/10.1007/978-3-031-05774-8_2

understanding, this presupposes perfect information and knowledge about the interests of all actors involved. The "homo economicus", who has complete knowledge of his environment, a stable set of preferences, and the ability to weigh among available alternatives to choose the course of action that best suits his preferences, has received much criticism for being too abstract to represent the actual behavior of intendedly rational individuals in particular circumstances. Indeed, this presents a debate as to whether normative or positive claims should be inherent in theories (March, 1978).

Following this critique, the scholarly literature in economics and public policy soon gathered under the common label of bounded rationality (B. D. Jones, 1999; Simon, 1955). Essential in this debate was the work of Herbert A. Simon, who received the Nobel Prize in 1978 for his work on the behavior of actors in organizations (Simon, 1947, 1955, 1978, 1985, 1990). A behavioral model of rationality, they argued, that models real behavior is based on bounded rationality. Rationality is bounded when there are constraints on the completeness of information, the definition of a problem, or the cognitive abilities and/or resources of individual agents to choose among alternative solutions to the problem, distinguishing between different roots of boundedness (Forester, 1984). The model takes into account imperfect information and uncertainty when making rational decisions, while at the same time granting policy actors the ability to learn from mistakes made (i.e., irrational decisions) (March, 1978; Simon, 1955).

In contemporary policy process research, bounded rationality is a frequently received psychological foundation for the behavior of policy actors. Scholars even speak of a behavioral turn in policy sciences (Leong & Howlett, 2020). Challenging the assumption of individual rationality, the Advocacy Coalition Framework (ACF) draws on the psychological concept of belief systems to explain collective action and the formation of advocacy coalitions through shared policy core beliefs (Calanni et al., 2014; Jenkins-Smith et al., 2017; Sabatier & Brasher, 1993). Building on this, the Narrative Policy Framework (NPF), developed only earlier this century, approaches collective action through the use of coherent policy narratives (Gupta et al., 2018; Shanahan et al., 2017). Other policy process frameworks focus on situational occasions exploited by policy entrepreneurs (Multiple Streams Framework, MSF) (Herweg et al., 2017) or on changing attention to policy issues that lead to major policy change (Baumgartner et al., 2017). None of these approaches place an explicit focus on the role of biographies or social identities in explaining collective action, which is what the PAF contributes to explaining policy change and stability. The subsequent chapters will delineate the PAF and embed it in the current state of research according to three main lines: cognitive foundations of policy actors' motivations, drivers of collective action, and mechanisms leading to policy change.

2.1   SOCIAL GROUPS, BIOGRAPHIES, AND POLICY PROGRAMS

In France, the role of a dominant and powerful public bureaucracy (Rouban, 1989, p. 45; Vernardakis, 2013) and a strong executive due to the semi-presidential system (Keeler, 1993) led to the emergence of a theoretical perspective called the programmatic approach (Genieys & Hassenteufel, 2012). This seeks the roots of policy change in the cooperation of actors close to the state who have similar career trajectories and promote a common policy program over several years. They do this to advance their careers, increase their authority, and realize their policy ideas.

Following these observations, the PAF postulates the argument that individual actors close to the state administration form programmatic groups based on shared biographical experiences. These actors include—among others—bureaucrats and actors from self-governance. Programmatic groups function as social groups and are committed to promoting a joint policy program. A programmatic group encompasses programmatic actors who are hypothesized to coalesce on the basis of shared biographical identities and have direct access to the state's policy-making apparatus. They are called programmatic actors because they subscribe to a shared policy program that is nameable and on which the programmatic actors agree. This can either be explicit, such as the creation of a document or the name of a group that meets regularly under the same label. Or the program may be implicit in the sense that asking each programmatic actor about their program would lead to highly overlapping results in the formulation. A policy program is defined as a set of policy goals and policy instruments that follow a consensus view of problems and solutions and focus on a particular policy sector. The individual policy reforms represent steps toward implementing the programmatic vision, but they are linked by the common policy goals articulated in the policy program. The immediate first incentive to join a programmatic group is strategic, as programmatic actors associate it with the prospect of advancing their own careers. Following on from this, there is a second, normative, and psychologically based impulse that drives individual policy actors to engage in collective action: a shared view of problems and solutions in a given policy sector, rooted in biographical association with the other programmatic actors and the resulting social identity.

Drawing on elite sociology, it is the career paths and biographies that led a group of scholars around Genieys, Hassenteufel, and Smyrl to formulate the programmatic approach as an alternative perspective on policy processes (Genieys & Hassenteufel, 2001; Genieys & Smyrl, 2008c). The insight that decision-making processes are shaped by a multitude of elites acting in the policy process is not limited to France, but also eminent in German elite research (von Beyme, 2001). Based on the analysis of French policy processes, the "approche programmatique" (French for programmatic approach) finds an endogenous explanation for policy change in the trajectories of policy elites and their policy programs (Genieys & Hassenteufel, 2012, p. 3). Endogenous in that they see policy change as the result of ongoing competition among elite actors and career-seeking individuals within the state (Genieys & Smyrl, 2008c, p. 90). In particular, the homogeneity of trajectories was seen as a key driver for collaboration and the resulting influence on decision-making processes. To specify this, the publication by Genieys and Smyrl (2008b) contains both theoretical assumptions and mechanisms as well as the first empirical case studies that demonstrate the existence of what the authors call programmatic elites. These programmatic elites are described as "a group of actors with direct access to policy-making positions that is self-consciously structured around a common commitment to a concrete and coherent programmatic model for a given policy sector" (Genieys & Smyrl, 2008c, p. 76).

Regarding the underlying assumptions and motives of individuals on which the theoretical mechanisms of programmatic elite competition with resulting policy change are based, Genieys and Smyrl (2008a) discuss these predispositions intensively and place them in the broader realm of bureaucratic theory, micro-level motivations for the pursuit of policy change, and the types of actors that a programmatic elite can encompass. In it, the pursuit of legitimate authority (p. 29) is seen as driving some— but by no means all—policy actors with direct access to the decision-making process, that is, those who directly formulate laws and regulations or have direct access to those who do. Their preferences are described as flexible to some degree (p. 30), and their rationality is assumed only insofar as it involves the pursuit of legitimate authority (p. 44).

While the policy program and the programmatic elite are mutually reinforcing, it is unclear whether the program precedes the elite group that gathers around it (Genieys & Michel, 2005, p. 187) or whether the group exists before its program is developed. One can bluntly argue that this is a question of empirics rather than theory, as theoretical considerations are primarily concerned with what drives successful programmatic action and under what conditions it occurs. Thus, it may be both that a programmatic group forms around an existing policy idea or that it emerges before it formulates its policy program.

Indeed, looking at career trajectories and "life cycles" (Michel, 2008, p. 165) in the study of programmatic elites might lead us to consider related concepts of generational change not only in policy processes (Obinger, 2012), but also in terms of the values and attitudes that different generations exhibit (Fisher, 2020; Shaykhutdinov, 2019; Wu & Lin, 2019). Generational change, however, implies a compelling exchange of generations as a function of elapsed time, regardless of how a particular group's positions change, how its policy program changes, or how networks are built and dissolved. Consequently, what is captured by a consideration of generations is not the focus of the programmatic approach.

Already in the early versions of the programmatic approach, there is a reference to programmatic elites as social groups, their sectoral meaning, and corresponding identity (Genieys, 2010, p. 14). In particular, the emphasis on programmatic actors coalescing into social groups and social identities driving the group dynamics of these actors to explain their collective action in the policy process has been the subject of ongoing reinterpretation and development of the PAF. This represents the only recent starting point for incorporating social identities in the policy process (Hornung, Bandelow & Vogeler, 2019).

In an attempt to integrate psychological and social psychological insights into the study of public administration and public policy, new strands of research have emerged under the labels of Behavioral Public Administration (Bhanot & Linos, 2019; Grimmelikhuijsen et al., 2017) and Behavioral Public Policy (Ewert, 2019; John & Stoker, 2019; Lodge, 2019; Strassheim, 2019). The concepts of bounded rationality have long been part of policy process research and, in particular, actor-centered theories of the policy process assume a model of the individual from which psychological assumptions allow the derivation of behavioral hypotheses.

In contrast, social identity theories have found little entry into policy process research, but their disregard is considered an "enormous blind spot" (Béland, 2019, p. 29). Far better known in political science are the big five personality traits of extraversion, agreeableness, conscientiousness, emotional stability, and intellect/imagination (Goldberg, 1990; McCrae & Costa, 1987), which are increasingly referenced in research on political behavior (Ackermann, 2016; Duckitt & Sibley, 2016; Weinschenk, 2017). However, these are difficult to operationalize for policy actors relevant to policy processes. Questionnaires tend to be extensive, and even the brief measures of personality traits rely on 10-item measures (Gosling et al., 2003), which are unlikely to be fully answered by a sufficient number of policy actors. It should not be neglected here that the big five personality traits may be able to shed light on important behavioral observations of policy actors, for example, how high levels of extraversion and agreeableness make policy actors more likely to engage in policy entrepreneurship (Timmermans et al., 2014, pp. 5-6). However, addressing how policy actors work together and how collective action leads to policy change suggests a more social psychological integration of psychological insights in the form of social identity research.

Compared to existing psychological foundations for policy process theories, the Social Identity Approach (SIA) offers a complementary theoretical perspective on individual preferences and behavior. The SIA circumscribes the combination of the Social Identity Theory (SIT) and the Self-Categorization Theory (SCT). The former was developed largely by Tajfel (1974) and the latter was refined by his student Turner (1982) (Hornsey, 2008, p. 208). Their approaches are interrelated and both relate to the concept of social groups, albeit with slightly different emphases. Originally developed as a theory of intergroup relations, the SIT seeks to examine intergroup behavior to explain cooperation and conflict between groups, focusing on in-group and out-group behavior, and the behavior that individuals exhibit in intergroup relations. Here, Tajfel defines social identity as "that part of the individual's self-concept which derives from their knowledge of their membership of a s social group (or groups) together with the value and emotional significance attached to that membership" (Tajfel, 1982, p. 3). The SCT is more concerned with the intragroup processes and cognitive aspects of identification and aims to uncover the underlying cognitive processes of individuals as they assign themselves and others to social categories and behave accordingly. The cognitive processes that lead individuals to identify with a social group are the parallel desires for sameness and distinction, summarized in a model of optimal distinctiveness (Brewer, 1991). A social identity consists of a triad of cognitive and affective components articulated as belongingness, positive evaluation, and emotional attachment (Tajfel, 1978, p. 372).

Although political science has adopted identity concepts from psychological research, not all of these identity concepts are related to the SIA (Weiner & Tatum, 2020), or the identity theory as part of the self-concept besides and apart from social identity (Hogg et al., 1995). Those that are related to the SIA use social identities as a refinement of already familiar concepts, such as partisanship (Greene, 1999, 2004). Conceptualizing partisanship as a social identity allows for examining the dynamics of partisan polarization (Iyengar & Westwood, 2015). At a micro level, Goren (2005) outlines how party group membership shapes core values and preferences, rather than party group membership being the result of preexisting core values and preferences. Party group members have been shown to be more attached to the party as a group than to what the party stands for, and to remain loyal to the party even when issues, platforms, and leaders change, which has been described as expressive rather than instrumental partisanship (Huddy et al., 2015, p. 15). This holds true in multiparty systems (Bankert et al., 2016). Nevertheless, this relation is still the subject of controversial findings and ongoing research (Egan, 2019)

Others relate the identity concept to the influence of peer networks and friends on preferences and behavior, for example when the salience of partisan identities depends on the party affiliation of friends (Parsons, 2015, p. 681). In these cases, social group membership is also associated with social pressures that lead individuals to follow group norms (Gerber et al., 2008). Other examples include when the online political behavior of individuals with high belongingness needs is influenced by whether their friends engage in online political activity (Bäck et al., 2020), or when personal friendships of actors in city governments determine the extent to which information is shared across those governments (Ki et al., 2020, p. 23).

In view of the need in policy process research to develop alternative models of the individual beyond rational choice (Millar et al., 2019, p. 114), Hornung et al. (2019) transfer the perspective of social identities to explain the behavior of policy actors in the policy process. A novelty here lies in the assumption that preferences and behavior are not antecedent but descendent of group memberships and that the thinking and behavior of group members converge over time and gain cohesion.

Hornung et al. (2019) distinguish five macro-level identities that can be salient in policy processes and are attributed to the following different social groups in the political arena:

- any type of policy-related organization, including political party groups (Bartle & Bellucci, 2009);
- any type of group related to the region or locality to which the individuals belong. This refers to the conflict between subnational and national levels of policy-making (Hildebrandt & Trüdinger, 2020) but also to geographical affiliations of place (Devine-Wright & Howes, 2010) or supranational, more abstract identities such as European identities (Kuhn & Nicoli, 2020);
- sectoral groups that emerge from sectoral professionalization and ongoing sectoral collaboration on a particular topical issue (Eriksson, 2017), and resulting policy styles (Padgett, 1990);
- demographic and biographical identities that involve an individual's early socialization through education and work experience, but also less formalized life experiences and biographical events;
- informal groups in the policy process, consisting of an informal collaboration familiar from the US Congress (Stevens et al., 1981) and other parliaments (Osei & Malang, 2016; Steinert & Yordanova, 2016).

The definition of social groups thereby follows Turner's as "two or more individuals who share a common social identification of themselves or, which is nearly the same thing, perceive themselves to be members of the same social category" (Turner, 1982, p. 15) and the important observation that "members of a social group seem often to share no more than a collective perception of their own social unity and yet this seems to be sufficient for them to act as a group" (Turner, 1982, p. 15). In considering these types of identities, the role of demographic identities in particular emerged as not being adequately addressed in current policy process research.

What need to be considered when applying the theoretical perspective of social identities to policy process research are the professional identities of policy actors. Aschhoff and Vogel (2019, p. 715) note that working in collaborative projects can establish a shift from professional identities to an identity created through collaboration. Similarly, agreements can create a shared identity by institutionalizing values that provide an anchor for identification (Duina, 2019). Given the multiplicity of existing social identities, their use as a valuable adjunct to explain behavior in the political sphere raises several key challenges, among the most important of which is defining the boundaries of political groups (Huddy, 2001, p. 145). In order for groups to be clearly delineated and for individuals to clearly identify the boundaries of the in-group versus the out-group, it is imperative that the group has identifying features such as a group name (Ren et al., 2012, p. 847). A second challenge relates to determining which identities actually matter in the policy process, that is, which are salient and strong, and what happens when the social identification with a group no longer leads to positive ingroup perceptions of distinction. The issue of identity salience is particularly relevant under different context-specific conditions (Vogeler, Hornung & Bandelow, 2020). Different ways of dealing with negative feelings of identity include not only leaving the group, but also changing the reference base for comparison with other groups and actively trying to change status hierarchies and intragroup dynamics (Hornsey, 2008, p. 207).

In short, the core argument of social identity in policy process research is that social identification with a group arises from the cooperation of actors who initially form a group and that individual preferences and behavior are guided by social identities. In the case of multiple identities, the salience of an identity depends on institutional circumstances as well as the strength of the social identity.

According to the flow diagram shown in Fig. 2.1, institutional opportunities and constraints influence the entire process of programmatic action. Programmatic action is defined as an instance in which programmatic groups successfully form and pursue their policy program to the ultimate outcome of policy change. This process is characterized by several steps that correspond to hypotheses about group formation and the success of programmatic groups and policy programs.

Briefly summarized, the model begins at the bottom with the entire field of policy actors in their "natural state", that is, they are policy actors with different social identities (since each individual is member in multiple social groups) but do not (yet) have a programmatic identity, since there are no programmatic groups. These actors follow a duality of incentives in their behavior: a rational motive to advance their careers and authority (what to achieve), and an ideational motive to normatively shape policies (how to achieve it). Some of these policy actors already hold positions and resources of moderate importance because they began careers in one of

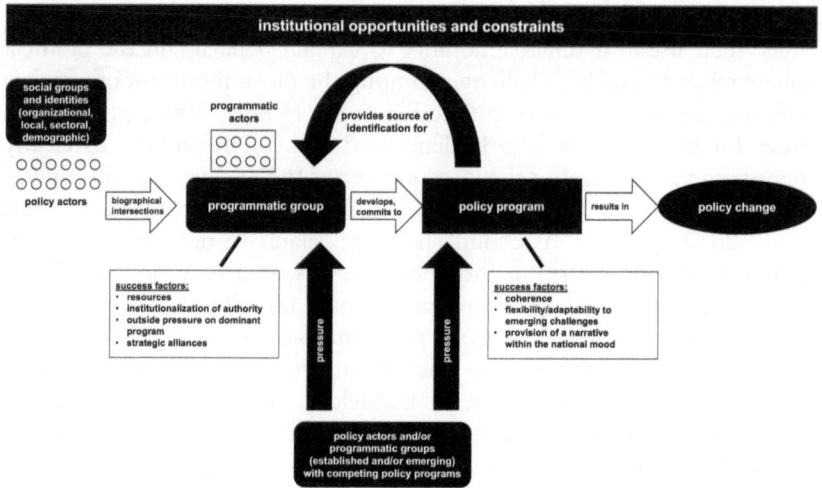

Fig. 2.1   The programmatic action framework. Source: Slightly modified on the basis of Bandelow, Hornung, and Smyrl (2021, p. 11)

the sectoral associations or were recruited through party-political channels. At some point, they may (but do not necessarily) coalesce into programmatic groups to further their goals. This is hypothesized to happen if there are homogeneous career paths, biographical linkages, and institutionalized or informal venues of exchange. Once there is a programmatic group, this social group forms a social identity of programmatic actors and at the same time commits itself to a policy program, which binds the group together and further strengthens social identification. Thus, a previous biographical identity then becomes a programmatic identity (no programmatic group exists without a program, and no program exists without programmatic actors). The program is thus an expression of the ideational positions of the programmatic actors and an instrument for achieving their goals. The success factors for the programmatic group and its policy program that ultimately help them achieve policy change lie in the programmatic group's ability to spread its ideas, institutionalize them, form alliances, or use the breaking of existing alliances to its advantage.

In the step-by-step description of the mechanisms inherent in this theoretical model, it becomes clear that one element in the PAF is still undertheorized and its influence on programmatic action is not yet sufficiently differentiated. This is the case with institutional opportunities. As a result, although empirical applications of the PAF already exist, they rarely address the institutions that enable or hinder programmatic action. Instead, they are merely points of contact or indications of potentially relevant institutions, such as the particular importance of self-governance in German health policy (Hornung & Bandelow, 2020). Hassenteufel et al. (2010) provide a starting point by arguing that variations in institutional settings influence the types of programmatic actors one is likely to find. However, they do not focus on the similarity of institutional settings that enable programmatic action in the first place. Bringing these institutions together with the study of policy process research is an attempt that has been successfully made by other theoretical frameworks (Fischer, 2015; Lubell, 2003; Wenzelburger, 2015; Zohlnhöfer et al., 2016). This study intends to do the same for the PAF, asking about the very institutions in different states that enable or hinder programmatic action.

Policy actors refer to those actors who are directly involved in policy-making. Assuming that policy actors seek authority in competition with other policy actors, cooperate with other policy actors based on shared biographies, and normatively use a policy program to achieve their strategic goal, the social group resulting from this mechanism is referred to as a programmatic group. Programmatic groups are thus defined as social groups that form around a policy program and thus form a social identity. Their members join together on the basis of biographical ties, pursue a strategic and an ideational goal, the latter being a means to achieve the former (Saurugger, 2013), and commit to the group's policy program to this end. When policy actors form programmatic groups, they become programmatic actors.

The concept of policy programs differs from existing conceptualizations of policy content in policy process research. A policy program is defined as not only arguments, measures, and instruments of policy change to achieve specific policy goals, but also a shared strategy in doing, so as well as a previously shared view of existing policy failures and problems (Hassenteufel & Genieys, 2021). Due to its visionary nature, programmatic change in policy sectors is often only visible after several years, when first steps of the program have been implemented and a coherent vision can be observed in the adopted reforms. In this respect, it is comparable to a so-called institutionalized reform that is implemented gradually and planned as a learning, adaptive system (Pannowitsch, 2009, p. 142). Nevertheless, observing innovative impulses in a policy sector that have the potential to shape it over several years and that are tied to a group of actors who publicly relate to the idea of the policy program and are biographically bound always allows for speculation about possible future policy programs.

Policy programs differ from policy paradigms, regimes, and alternatives (Hall, 1993; Howlett et al., 2006; Wilson, 2000) in two major respects. Firstly, a policy program is associated with a programmatic group. While policy paradigms, regimes, and alternatives may be promoted by collective actors such as collective policy entrepreneurs (Stephenson, 2010, p. 730), and policy entrepreneurs may also make a policy alternative to their pet policy, these connections are not hypothesized to be driven by social identities, nor are they based on biographical intersections between the actors. The PAF assumes that a programmatic group is a social group that creates its own social identity and uses as a defining element of the group the policy program to which it commits. Through social identification, individual members are guided in their behavior by the norms and values of the programmatic group, which, unlike in the ACF's understanding, do not come from beliefs developed through socialization but are handed down by the social group.

Secondly, a policy program is an instrument in the power struggle between competing policy actors. It is not necessarily associated with a particular set of policy beliefs. However, actors tend to formulate programs that correspond to some of their values and attitudes. More important is the alignment of the policy program with the strategic goal of the social group, which is to gain authority within the sector in question. Policy programs are thus used by programmatic groups to gain power positions in the sector. The development, maintenance, or—in the case of new members joining the programmatic group—takeover of a policy program follows strategic individual interests. Competing policy programs may appeal to similar beliefs and values. Once a programmatic group establishes dominance of its policy program, it defends it not out of conviction or ideological beliefs, but because of inherent strategic interest, since the programmatic group's authority rests on the program's dominance. Individual members of the programmatic group have an interest in the stability of the program because it legitimizes the institutions that have emerged in the wake of the program and guarantees their authority.

The persistence of a policy program is explained by precisely this long-term social identification. Even if advocating a different policy is more beneficial to an individual in the short or long term than adhering to the policy program, social identity prevents rejection of the jointly developed program. Although a policy program is rarely a paradigm, since it need not provide a holistic view and need not state causal relations or assumptions, a paradigm can be used as a policy program if it is adopted for a defined subsystem. Policy programs are also much more explicitly linked to policy change than the current discussion of the relation between policy paradigms and policy change would suggest (Daigneault, 2014, p. 463).

2.2   AMBIGUITY AND MULTIPLE STREAMS IN THE POLICY PROCESS

Ambiguity and time are the key constraints on rational behavior in the MSF (Zohlnhöfer & Rüb, 2016). To cope with the complex environment in which policy actors find themselves, they not only engage in routines (Lindblom, 1959; Wildavsky, 1964) (Lindblom, 1959; Wildavsky, 1964) that would suggest incremental change, but their cognitive capacities force them to selective attention. As a result, policy actors may pay only serial attention to issues (Simon, 1985), with only one issue receiving the most attention. Analogously, the political system may consider only one issue at a time at the highest level of the political agenda. Originally developed to explain agenda setting, the MSF draws on this understanding of prioritization of attention to formulate hypotheses about how situational factors in an ambiguous environment promote a policy proposal to the top of the agenda. The core of this idea is found in the title "Agendas, Alternatives and Public Policies" by Kingdon (2003).

Rationality is bounded not only by the limited time available to actors to process information, but also by the phenomenon of ambiguity. The MSF assumes that the definition of problems and the solutions available to solve them are subject to ambiguity in the sense that they cannot be interpreted in a definite way but comprise different aspects that can be considered. A high degree of ambiguity among policy actors then leads to a situation in which many policy actors have no preconceived opinion on many policy issues and are therefore easily persuaded that a proposed policy measure is necessary or desirable at a particular time. Such a predisposition leads to the idea that situational aspects are crucial in the adoption of a policy. In developing the MSF, situational relevance was portrayed as a parallel flow of problem stream, policy stream, and politics or political stream, which has to be coupled by a policy entrepreneur when a window of opportunity opens. The problem stream includes problem definitions and matters of public attention; the policy stream entails possible policy solutions; the political stream consists of features that are elemental to everyday politics, such as the national mood, elections or changes in government, and interest groups (Béland & Howlett, 2016, p. 222; Zahariadis, 2003, 2016). By national mood, scholars often mean public opinion (Durr, 1993; Enns & Kellstedt, 2008), operationalized, for example, by the salience of certain issues to the public (Bromley-Trujillo & Poe, 2020). The particular pertinence of situations and entrepreneurs inherent in the MSF is informed by insights from organizational theory, particularly the garbage can model of organizational choice, which views solutions as floating independently of designated problems and emphasizes the chaotic, anarchistic nature of decision-making in organizations (Cohen et al., 1972). Criticisms of translating the garbage can model into an analytical frameworks call for more explicit consideration of the institutional context (Sætren, 2016, p. 27).

The application of the MSF has successfully answered this claim, translating the perspective from US-American politics to European policy process research and the EU (Ackrill et al., 2013; Herweg, 2016). In the course of assessing the traveling capacity of the MSF, several adaptations accompanied this endeavor. One is the adaptation of the MSF to parliamentary party systems with a particular focus on institutions (Herweg et al., 2015). Another concerns not only the application of the MSF to agenda-setting processes, but its extension to the decision-making process with a separate coupling process (Zohlnhöfer et al., 2016) or implementation (Fowler, 2018, 2020; Howlett, 2018). This includes the observation that in the agenda-setting stage, it is sufficient to generate interest among policy actors, while in the later stage of decision-making, it is necessary to organize the required majority for the adoption of the policy proposal (Zohlnhöfer, 2016). A consideration of the institutional conditions under which policy actors operate is not only important for the MSF studies on policy entrepreneurs, but indispensable for any theoretical perspective dealing with agency and actor behavior in the policy process. It is the essence of the connection between ideas and institutions.

In addition to the policy entrepreneur, other types of actors populate the current landscape of MSF research. Although the ontological underpinnings are different, advocacy coalitions can be integrated into the political stream, and epistemic communities and instrument constituencies have been theorized to be relevant in the problem and policy stream, respectively (Mukherjee & Howlett, 2015). It is in the political stream, at the decision-making stage, that a political entrepreneur can excel. By holding an elected position with formal decision-making power, the political entrepreneur is able to adopt an idea prepared by the policy entrepreneur in the policy stream and agenda-setting stage, increasing the likelihood of adoption depending on the veto players standing in their way (Herweg et al., 2015; Zohlnhöfer et al., 2016). Several case studies empirically confirm the notion of the political entrepreneur, such as research on labor market policy (Zohlnhöfer, 2016), infrastructure policy (Bandelow & Vogeler, 2019), local energy policy (Kagan, 2019), and administrative reforms (Lichtmannegger & Tobias, 2020). Other types of actors include the problem broker, who defines and frames problems in the problem stream and provides tying knots for the policy entrepreneur (Knaggård, 2015). In this context, what is ultimately considered a problem also depends on the institutional conditions of the dominant coalitions and networks (Reardon, 2018). Another is the "bricoleur", who takes responsibility for finding the best possible solution to a given problem, choosing from a variety of existing solutions and ideas (Carstensen, 2011, p. 154; Deruelle, 2016, p. 49).

Based on how agency is conceptualized in the MSF, an important aspect of interest here is what entrepreneurial strategies ensure the success of a policy proposal. A policy entrepreneur is a corporate or individual actor, for example, a rapporteur in the European Parliament (Thierse, 2019), who promotes a proposal in the policy stream to make it a notable alternative in the policy community (Herweg et al., 2017, p. 28). Together with resources and access to decision-makers, entrepreneurial strategies represent the key to entrepreneurial achievement (M. D. Jones et al., 2016, p. 16). Entrepreneurial strategies include bargaining, the use of narrative stories (Tullia Galanti & Sacchi, 2019) or other discursive strategies such as framing and issue linking (Zahariadis & Exadaktylos, 2016, p. 62f), the continuous formation of supportive coalitions (Mintrom & Norman, 2009), venue shopping (Brunner, 2008, p. 505), promoting their own expertise (Witting & Dudley, 2020), and "salami tactics", that is, dividing the effort into several phases and promoting a policy proposal stepwise (Zahariadis, 2003, p. 14f). By organizing themselves into smaller groups, policy entrepreneurs can also strategically prevent opposition actors from gaining access to decision-making processes in order to ensure their own success (Johannesson & Qvist, 2020, p. 4). *Thus, in their actions, entrepreneurs and policy actors are always enabled and constrained by institutions* (Zahariadis & Exadaktylos, 2016, p. 62). Recent research has also identified a type of institutional entrepreneurship that describes cases in which policy actors span multiple institutional contexts and draw inspiration for policy innovation and institutional change from them (Bakir & Jarvis, 2017, p. 466). There is evidence of the existence of Institutional entrepreneurs in health policy, for example, when actors with professional experience in a policy sector enter the policy-making process to bring their normative ideas to policy-makers and public officials (V. Smith & Cumming, 2017, p. 532). Drawing on the literature on knowledge utilization, Blum (2017) develops the concept of argumentative coupling, which describes the strategic use of scientific arguments and evidence to couple streams. The active role of the policy entrepreneur may even extend to influencing the opening of a policy window, especially at smaller levels of government (Cairney, 2018, p. 202). Such strategies for success may also be fruitful, at least in part, for other types of actors in the policy process, including programmatic groups.

With respect to the PAF, there are some parallels that can be drawn when comparing it to the MSF, and some blind spots that the PAF may fill. Kingdon's original book remains intentionally non-specific about the source of ideas, finding them "anywhere" (Béland, 2016, p. 231). By focusing on the emergence of policy programs, the PAF echoes this view, but sheds more light on how a policy program is composed from the multitude of existing ideas and how it is purposefully designed by intellectual circles. It thereby implies a much stronger linkage to the policy design literature (Capano & Lippi, 2017; Howlett et al., 2018; Peters et al., 2018). In this regard, the PAF's understanding of a programmatic group that deploys a policy program for strategic and normative purposes is compatible with the MSF's understanding of the motivational drivers of policy entrepreneurs. Kingdon finds these drivers in "self-interest, the promotion of values, passion for shaping policy, and the pleasure that advocacy and public exposure give them" (Béland, 2016, p. 233; Kingdon, 2003, p. 123). Moreover, programmatic groups resemble policy entrepreneurs in that they also link their policy solutions (policy programs) to a defined problem, whether framed by themselves or by problem brokers. MSF research could thus benefit from integrating the concept of programmatic groups as a specific type of entrepreneur with different resources and a more narrowly defined policy program. However, the important distinction of the PAF remains in the social psychological view of social groups and identities in the policy process. Programmatic groups are bound by the policy program, and their shared experience and resulting mutual trust ensures long-term cooperation among programmatic actors beyond purely rational interests. Thus, the longevity of programmatic action and reliance on long-term strategies and careers rather than situational opportunities for major policy change is the key distinguishing feature of the MSF and the PAF.

Given the often complex and historical nature of health care institutions, combining entrepreneurship and agency-based explanations for major reforms with institutional predispositions is critical to explaining policy outcomes (V. Smith & Cumming, 2017). The combination of the Multiple Streams Framework and institutional veto players (Zohlnhöfer, 2016, p. 89), as well as the MSF and historical institutionalism, in which policy entrepreneurs that use policy windows present critical junctures (Spohr, 2016) has proven fruitful. *This is close to the PAF's idea of linking individual actors with the institutional positions they hold and integrating both aspects into a coherent framework of policy change.* Following on from the roots of collective action, the next two subchapters turn attention to different types of groups, networks, and coalitions, both to highlight the limitations and hypotheses of programmatic groups and to work out the essence of programmatic groups compared to other types of networks.

2.3   BELIEFS AND ADVOCACY COALITIONS IN THE POLICY PROCESS

One of the most prominent and widely applied actor-centered frameworks in policy process research focused on networks is the ACF. Consistent with the line of thought that traces the psychological roots of actor-centered approaches in public policy, the ACF continues the understanding of a boundedly rational individual, but seeks the limits to rational processing of information not in ambiguity and time constraints, but in the existence of belief systems. Belief systems are cognitively existing sets of elements that collectively represent coherent individual attitudes, values, and preferences (Converse, 2006, p. 3). Explicitly following Converse, Sabatier adapted this understanding to elite belief systems, proposing that they encompass perceptions of causal mechanisms that relate to policy areas (Sabatier & Hunter, 1989). Accordingly, in the ACF, belief systems are defined as "sets of value priorities and causal assumptions about how to realize them" (Sabatier, 1988, p. 131). The notion that they are hierarchically structured into three levels, with (1) deep normative core beliefs,

(2) policy-related core beliefs, and (3) secondary aspects, is borrowed from Lakatos' conceptualization of scientific research programs (Jenkins-Smith et al., 2017, p. 136; Lakatos & Musgrave, 1970).

Over the past three decades, the conceptualization of belief systems has been both challenged and advanced (Brandt et al., 2019; Hann, 1995; Ripberger et al., 2014). In operationalizing deep normative core beliefs, Sabatier and Jenkins-Smith (1993) originally referred to basic convictions regarding the relation between nature and humans that were reinforced by socialization (Searing et al., 1973). However, this operationalization has been specified using cultural theory, which approaches them through the concepts of individualism, fatalism, egalitarianism, and hierarchy (Jenkins-Smith et al., 2014; M. D. Jones, 2011; Sotirov & Winkel, 2016). Underlying this research is the central research interest of what drives individual political preferences, with current explanations for political attitudes ranging from biological to partisan, cultural, and belief-driven (Bachner & Hill, 2014). Bachner and Hill (2014, p. S65) emphasize that further research is needed to specify under which conditions which factor is more relevant. Context and individually different ways of interpreting the world, caused either by belief systems or other types of cognitive filters, thus considerably shape the formation of policy preferences. Because belief systems influence how actors interpret and process information, actors are more susceptible to cognitive bias and differences in how they perceive the world and the information presented in it, leading to segregated policy networks (Henry, 2011a) and biased assimilation of policy preferences and policy beliefs (Moyson, 2017). Therefore, psychological and social psychological approaches to explaining individual preferences have proven insightful when integrated into the study of policy processes.

The contemporary understanding of the ACF largely runs along three lines—advocacy coalitions, policy change, and policy-oriented learning (Weible & Nohrstedt, 2012). Shared policy core beliefs present the unifying force of advocacy coalitions that strive to translate their policy preferences into adopted policies (Zafonte & Sabatier, 1998). An important element of cooperation among coalitions is the trust that follows from shared policy core beliefs, as well as from small and stable groups (Leach & Sabatier, 2005). Advocacy coalitions compete for dominance in a policy subsystem and use their collective resources to achieve policy change in the direction of their own policy preferences. Depending on the degree of cooperation between competing advocacy coalitions, policy-oriented learning becomes more or less likely (Koebele, 2018, p. 50). The defining characteristics of advocacy coalitions are that they consist of policy actors who share policy core beliefs, act in a coordinated manner, pool resources, and are stable over time (Weible et al., 2019).

For policy change to occur, the original ACF places a strong emphasis on the role of policy-oriented learning. Policy-oriented learning occurs when experiences and knowledge lead to the modification of beliefs or secondary aspects (Sabatier, 1987). However, there is an important distinction between minor change (change in secondary aspects) and major change (change in the policy core) in policies that has received less attention in ACF studies (Pierce et al., 2017, p. S29). Hypotheses expecting policy learning under conditions of forums, quantitative performance measures, and policy subsystems of natural sciences were added and modified, while the core assumptions defined above were left largely unchanged (Wellstead, 2017, p. 558). However, learning processes can also be the result of adaptive reactions to criticism in the absence of external shocks (Lertzman et al., 1996).

Meanwhile, research on learning has expanded beyond the boundaries of the ACF and is currently discussed as a stand-alone framework or theory (Dunlop & Radaelli, 2018). While learning and belief change are not of central interest to the theoretical development of the PAF, not least because of the fundamentally different understanding of how preferences are formed, one aspect in the learning literature appears to be transferable to the concept of social and programmatic groups, that of socialization (Dunlop & Radaelli, 2017, p. 313). Whenever policy actors enter new positions with new constraints on their daily actions or find themselves in new situations, including new memberships in groups to which they begin to belong, their values change and so do their preferences.

It is precisely this influence of social groups on individual preferences and behavior that allows the PAF to propose a group-theoretic explanation of policy change. This goes beyond the cooperation among individuals to translate their shared beliefs into adopted policies, which defines collaborative action as an ideologically driven act to achieve subjective goals. Instead, the PAF sees the group itself as the main generator and driver of ideas. Not only is it a resource in promoting policy, but the success of the group itself becomes the central goal of its members' engagement in policy-making.

In addition to learning, the ACF describes three other pathways to policy change. First, negotiated agreements can serve as a mediating element between advocacy coalitions and lead to major policy change (Metz et al., 2020). For negotiated agreements to be concluded, policy broker-age can be a critical determinant of success (Ingold, 2011). Second, internal shocks to the subsystem and external perturbations can trigger change in the subsystem. These latter two types of shocks are similar to what the MSF calls policy windows that open from the political (internal shock) or problem (external shock) stream. Empirical studies of the ACF often combine several of these pathways to identify policy learning and, in particular, the possibility of major policy change as more likely under the impact of external or internal shocks (Albright, 2011; Ardıç et al., 2015; Crow et al., 2018; Markard et al., 2016; Sandström et al., 2020). Negotiated agreements receive relatively little attention compared to learning and external events, but more than internal events and superior jurisdictions (Pierce et al., 2020, p. 71).

Regarding the roots of collective action, the ACF complements research by focusing on the role of shared beliefs as binding elements of coalitions or networks. However, the initial desire to engage in collective action is a rational one, as actors expect benefits from joining coalitions and the opportunity to realize their policy preferences (Schlager, 1995). Since Sabatier's original thinking, this has been grounded in the Theory of Reasoned Action (Ajzen & Fishbein, 1980), which was later developed into the Theory of Planned Behavior (Ajzen, 1991) Criticisms focus on the ACF's inability to explain collective action problems, to which it responded by integrating access to information (Yagci, 2019), repeated interaction, or interdependencies (Fenger & Klok, 2001) as factors to overcome these problems. In addition to shared policy beliefs, empirical evidence supports the claim that perceived actor influence contributes to building actor relationships (Weible, 2005, p. 471) and that the preexistence of organizational structures fosters the formation of advocacy coalitions (Kübler, 2001, p. 628). Schmid et al. (2019) combine the ACF with PFT to outline how policies influence the structures of and available resources of advocacy coalitions. Such a view corresponds well with the added value of PFT, seen in this book particularly in the way policies account for the resources and dominance of a dominant programmatic group.

While the ACF assumes shared policy core beliefs as a predisposition for coalition formation, this unilateral causal direction is controversial in the current state of the art on networks and attitude formation. Numerous empirical studies have confirmed that actors adopt political values, attitudes, and preferences from those with whom they regularly interact in social relationships, not that they form social relationships based on their preexisting views (Goren, 2005; Lazer et al., 2010; Mcpherson et al., 2001). The PAF presents an attempt to integrate social psychological research on the SIA into theories of the policy process to fill this gap (Hogg et al., 2017; Hornung et al., 2019). The proposition that preferences are shaped later than group membership and that social identities are a crucial explanation for policy actors' behavior is a major innovation that the PAF contributes to existing policy process research.

In terms of the role of institutions, the ACF incorporates into its flow diagram and theoretical model political opportunity structures, by which it understands the stable parameters of institutional settings (Nohrstedt et al., 2020, p. 71). Specifically, these are the ways in which institutions influence actors' belief systems and their resulting behavior (Lubell, 2003). In the research literature, these have been operationalized as consensus or majoritarian democracies and openness of the political system, and more concretely as federalism and corporatism (Kübler, 2001; Weible et al., 2009, p. 124). For example, the ACF certainly recognizes that corporatist structures shape advocacy coalitions differently than non-corporatist settings with regard to the actors involved (Gronow et al., 2019). Institutional settings can also facilitate policy change through advocacy coalitions if they provide forums or institutionalized venues where negotiated agreements are reached (Metz et al., 2020, p. 20). Despite these advances, scholars still call for more research to identify the political institutions that actually matter for coalition-building (Heikkila et al., 2019, p. 163). Importantly, institutions can also change within subsystems and thereby influence coalition behavior, which Gupta (2014, p. 360) attributes at least in part to the role of political parties. The institutions included in ACF research therefore are similar to those analyzed in this study.

2.4   Network Theory and Agency in the Policy Process

Within the broader field of policy process research, there exist several theories about the formation of networks and their influence on policy-making. Since the notion of a programmatic group is comparable to a closely collaborating network, it is worthwhile to place PAF in the realm of network theories and to demarcate programmatic groups as a very specific type of network. Several studies have provided an overview of what can be considered a network and the different types of networks (Carlsson, 2000; G. Jordan & Schubert, 1992). Essential to any network conceptualization is the assumption about what drives individuals to engage in collaboration and joint action. A review of the MSF and ACF literature has highlighted the strategic use of alliances (as in the MSF) and the formation of coalitions around shared policy core beliefs to translate them into policy (as in the ACF) as potential motivations for individuals to collaborate with other policy actors. This chapter will consider a selection of the remaining types of networks, extrapolate their boundaries, and relate them to the new type of network, the programmatic group.

In order to use the concept of actor networks in policy process research, it is essential to adequately define their scope. This is most easily done by answering the following four questions: What actors does the network consist of, or can it theoretically consist of? Why do these actors work together, what is their motivation for joining the network? What holds the network together (the question is related to the decision of individuals to join a network, but the answer is not necessarily the same)? What is the goal of the network and what strategies are available? In reviewing the existing notions of networks that are prominently used in public policy research, these four answers are kept in mind to answer. While the literature on networks differs on whether individual actors or corporate actors, usually organizations, are the nodes within a network, when applying psychological explanations of collective action and group (or network) formation, the unit of analysis must logically be an individual. As a consequence, network theories that focus on corporate actors such as organizations are excluded from consideration, while acknowledging the extensive research on corporate actors such as the organizational state (Laumann & Knoke, 1987).

In policy process research, network theories are typically concerned with the study of elites. While there are several elite theories in other disciplines such as sociology (Rahman Khan, 2012; Scott, 2008), the study of policy networks dates back to C. Wright Mills' work on national power elites in the US to outline the importance of occupying key institutional positions in influencing the policy process in general and decision-making in particular (Knoke & Kostiuchenko, 2017, pp. 92-93; Mills, 2000, p. 9). Accordingly, most theories of the policy process explicitly designate the types of actors that are potentially of interest or subject to their theoretical propositions. In this regard, most policy process theories use the policy subsystem as the level of analysis (Nowlin, 2011, p. 54). The ACF has a fairly broad understanding of policy actors as those who populate a subsystem. Policy subsystems are distinguished as systems of specialized policy actors who engage with and seek to influence the policy issue (Sabatier & Weible, 2007, p. 192). Other ACF studies refer to it as "a partition of a broader governing system that focuses on a policy topic within a geographical area and involves specialized policy actors attempting to influence policy subsystem affairs" (Olofsson et al., 2018, pp. 645-646). The concept of policy subsystems overlaps with that of policy domains in that it encompasses public and private actors that revolve around a commonly perceived (policy) problem and are characterized by a shared desire to solve it (Laumann et al., 1985, p. 2).

In addition to the policy subsystem, other conceptualizations of networks and aggregates of actors have emerged. Rhodes refers to them all as policy networks (Roderick A. W. Rhodes, 2008, p. 425f). What they all have in common is a policy-oriented clustering of actors (corporate and/ or individual) and the description and analysis of their interconnections, especially those of state versus non-state (above all industrial) actors, with respect to their influence on policy-making processes. In this context, they denote a type of sectoral policy-making and are often understood as running along a continuum (Miller & Demir, 2007, p. 140). The terminological confusion and overlap of concepts also stem in part from the fact that some terminologies emerged from US contexts and empirical research on US politics and others are explicitly communicated from a British perspective, for example, policy communities (Roderick A. W. Rhodes, 1990, p. 302).

Howlett and Ramesh (1998, p. 469) distinguish between policy communities and policy networks, with the former encompassing a large set of actors who have knowledge of a policy topic and the latter comprising only those who collaborate out of an interest in influencing policy-making; both are seen as subsets of policy subsystems. Exactly how the concepts relate to each other, however, is a matter of debate in the research literature. While some agree with Howlett and Ramesh and see policy communities as broader than policy networks, with networks explicitly referring to the connections between actors, others see policy communities as a specific type of network (M. M. Atkinson & Coleman, 1992, p. 158). Policy communities are generally referred to as being limited—and therefore tantamount to—policy subsystems and sectors. Comparable to subgovernments, they are characterized by shared attitudes and temporally stable relationships between government groups in bureaucracy and politics and interest groups (G. Jordan, 1990, p. 331f). Because they are so exclusive, they promote exchange between members (Grant & MacNamara, 1995, p. 509). In doing so, they can also be territorially bound (Keating et al., 2009, p. 53), transnationally active (Stone, 2008), or competing in policy arenas for policy change (Dudley & Richardson, 1996). The terminological derivation of policy communities is essentially rooted in the critique of iron triangles and sub-governments as overly simplistic and exclusive representations of policy-making processes (G. Jordan & Maloney, 1997, pp. 559-561). This discussion dates back to the seminal work of Freeman and Stevens (1987) and concerns the early use of the term "policy subsystem", which was later opened up to include actors with specialized interests, making it issue-driven rather than actor-driven (McGee & Jones, 2019, pp. S140-142). Nonetheless, a conceptualization of policy communities allows for the emergence of subgroups such as advocacy coalitions (Birkland, 1998, p. 57).

In a similarly issue-driven perspective, the concept of issue networks, originally introduced by Heclo (1978), refers to the linkages between actors in a fragmented and highly diversified web of relationships among actors that influence policy-making. Freeman and Stevens (1987, p. 14) place them on a par with subsystems because of their vagueness in designating members. Unlike Rhodes' network perspective, Heclo sees members of issue networks as less bound and fixed, but floating, and the main motivation of actors is emotional or intellectual advancement rather than interests (Schneider, 2015, p. 375). Consequently, issue networks are much more open to actors who are not institutionally linked to the state, allowing them to be conceived as shapers of public policy, such as non-profit policy activists (Nyland, 1995). They are specifically tied to an issue, although they may differ in terms of their agreement on the concreteness of legislation, advocacy arguments, and conceptualization of the issue, as well as membership, member-to-member exchanges, and leadership (Kirst et al., 1984). In contrast to iron triangles and the neo-corporatist picture of policy-making, issue networks are less likely to resolve conflicts among their members than the latter, but more open than the former, with iron triangles limited to the presence of interest groups, and corresponding administrative and legislative bodies (A. G. Jordan, 1981, pp. 96-98). Within issue networks, evidence suggests that past experiences with network interactions also influence whether alliances will form in the future and that those who have had contact in the past are more likely to contact again compared to other actors in the same larger network (Heaney, 2004). As the network changes, so do the terms used to describe it. For example, M. J. Smith (1991) noted that as scandals and media attention on the issue of salmonella in eggs increased, the policy community morphed into an issue network, taking in actors who did not originally deal with this policy issue on a regular basis.

Similarly revolving around an expertise on a policy issue, but much narrower in scope than issue networks, epistemic communities include scientific experts on a policy issue. Originally introduced by Haas, the concept of "networks of knowledge-based experts" (Haas, 1992, p. 2) builds on the argument that state actors in contexts of uncertainty and complex policy problems form preferences based on the advice and knowledge integration of these epistemic communities. Therein lies their influence on the policy process. As they disseminate their knowledge, epistemic communities can cross national boundaries and shape international views that are translated into policies and treaties (Adler, 1992). Going beyond this initial narrow definition is the observation that policy actors with a biographical trajectory relevant to the issue at hand can be recruited by epistemic communities in the process of forming a strategic alliance to advance a policy proposal. In the case analyzed by Grødem and Hippe (2019), civil servants from the Norwegian Ministry of Finance formed an epistemic community and strategically cooperated with the prime minister, whose expertise was similar to theirs due to his educational background in economics. Alternatively, epistemic communities may also support advocacy coalitions, thereby impeding policy-oriented learning and a change in preferences based on incoming scientific information (Meijerink, 2005, p. 1070). In this context, which knowledge is provided by which epistemic communities is highly dependent on the respective policy actors. For example, the way international organizations such as the OECD and the World Bank select epistemic communities and draw on their knowledge depends on the mission pursued and the internal structures of the organization (Francesco & Guaschino, 2020, p. 115).

Policy communities, policy subsystems, sub-governments, iron triangles, issue networks—they all have a special focus on relationships between groups of actors and thus concern the meso level of action. While they often start from the policy issue before deriving the actors involved, they consider not only the structural setting of actors but also their interactions and influence on policy processes. In addition, they usually allow for the inclusion of interest groups and other actors who do not have formal institutional power to be relevant to the policy process. In considering individual action, many network approaches thereby look for the reasons why individual actors cooperate in interest-driven behavior—or do not specify the psychological basis for micro-level decisions to join networks at all. Moreover, interest-based action is usually an expression of rational behavior. However, there are other roots for collective action that explain cooperation in the absence of rational cost-benefit analyses. The PAF complements these perspectives by looking at biographies and career ambitions as drivers of collaboration and by integrating social identities.

A rather newer strand of research focuses on the concept of instrument constituencies. As the term implies, they are particularly concerned with one policy instrument and how it has been innovated and developed over the course of the policy process. This also means that they are not tied to one subsystem but span multiple policy cycles (Weible, 2018, p. 63). Despite obvious overlaps with the concept of epistemic communities, due to the focus on shared and exchanged knowledge and ideas, as well as a potential transnationality, Zito (2018) finds considerable differences between instrument constituencies, which are centered around and exist through the policy instrument, and the more knowledge-oriented epistemic community. However, both concepts include the possibility that their defining feature may become a source of shared group identity (Zito, 2018, p. 44). Following the MSF perspective of policy-making structured around the problem stream, the policy stream, and the politics stream, Béland, Howlett, and Mukherjee (2018, pp. 7-8) situate instrument constituencies in the policy stream because they develop and promote the solutions to which problems can be assigned and then because the promotion of those very solutions is their binding element. Consequently, the bond between the instrument constituency and the policy instrument it promotes may be so strong that one does not exist without the other, thus providing an important source of identification (Voß & Simons, 2014, p. 738). Interestingly, the concept of instrument constituencies also holds the structural promise that the implementation of a policy instrument may entail an increased demand for expertise and the creation of instrument-specific institutions, from which promoters of that instrument may benefit career-wise by occupying new positions (Simons & Voß, 2018, p. 22). This aspect is quite close to the career-related motivation of programmatic actors, but programmatic groups, in contrast to instrument constituencies, initially turn out to be rooted differently and characterized by a higher degree of cooperation and social identity.

Often, the alternative theoretical explanations outlined above share the argument that cooperation is a result of (or influences in a reciprocal way) some sort of sameness and cohesion among individuals. This sameness and cohesion can stem from similar cultural worldviews (Weare et al., 2014), ideology and policy core beliefs as in the ACF (Henry, 2011b), expert knowledge as in epistemic communities (Adler & Haas, 1992), issue-specific knowledge in issue networks (Kalafatis et al., 2015), coming together around specific policy design elements (Haelg et al., 2020, p. 331) or other characteristics shared by the actors. Narratives can also emerge as a unifying element of networks, referred to as narrative networks or discourse coalitions (R. Atkinson et al., 2011; Bulkeley, 2000; Ingram et al., 2019; Lejano et al., 2017). While sameness contributes to network integration, efficiency (in the sense of mobilizing resources to influence policy-making) and innovation in network activities grow from heterogeneity of actors in what regards their positions and resources (Sandström & Carlsson, 2008).

Based on a summary of several network approaches, the theory of collaborative policy networks proceeds starts the main defining features of networks to propose hypotheses about structural signatures of policy networks. For example, it states that collaborative policy networks are more likely to be characterized by diversity, reciprocity, horizontal power structures, long relationship histories, trust, transparent decision-making processes, and structurally equivalent leadership (DeLeon & Varda, 2009). The role of trust and reciprocity in particular is emphasized by theories of social capital, most prominently by Putnam's work "Bowling Alone", which proposes to define social capital as "features of social organization such as networks, norms, and social trust that facilitate coordination and cooperation for mutual benefit" (Putnam, 1995, p. 67). In public policy, social capital and trust have been studied in relation to how to overcome problems of collective action and management of common pool resources. Factors seen as contributing to mutual trust include: frequent interactions (Lubell, 2007, p. 248), cohesion among group members in terms of similar beliefs (Leach & Sabatier, 2005, p. 493; Lubell, 2007, p. 239; Parsons, 2020, p. 39), opportunities for and experiences with cooperation and collaboration (Fischer & Sciarini, 2015, p. 65), professional competence and expertise (Calanni et al., 2014, p. 917), resources, and power derived from network centrality (Berardo, 2008, pp. 186-187). From a psychological perspective, biased perceptions of opponents as more evil and powerful reduce trust (Fischer et al., 2016, p. 330) as do personal and individual predispositions that make it easier for certain individuals to trust others (Dinesen et al., 2014; Freitag & Bauer, 2016, p. 141). Research findings suggest that trust is a mandatory prerequisite for long-term close collaboration and that frequency of contact and commonalities foster trust. This comes closest to the idea of the PAF.

The development of the study of policy networks also contributes to research on institutions and public administration. Firstly, it also reveals the replacement of the long-held dichotomous view of politics and administration, in which bureaucrats are seen as purely functionally driven individuals directed by their respective political superiors (Skok, 1995, pp. 329-330). Instead, in the policy networks studied here, bureaucrats and administrative actors themselves can actively participate in the meaningful construction of agendas and the formulation and adoption of policies. Second, with respect to institutions, the argument that the institutional positions of policy actors and their structural positions in a network determine the perceived power of actors is underscored (Ingold & Leifeld, 2014). Overall, this confirms the added value of the PAF perspective, which also addresses these aspects.

Summarizing perspectives on policy networks and typologies of aggregates of policy actors, it is clear that an important prerequisite for comparing and advancing research is to be clear about the terms one uses to label one's work on policy actors. Depending on the scientific community in which research is conducted, different terms have different meanings and, accordingly, different assumptions about actors are predefined. Rather than getting caught up in trying to define structural limitations of subsystems, "it may be more fruitful to focus instead on the functional characteristics of subsystems, what is their behavior under specific conditions" (McCool, 1998, p. 558). This means that in choosing an appropriate term to describe the object of research, attention is drawn to how and what kinds of conflicts arise in policy-making processes and how they are constrained by existing conditions. Similarly, it is important to be clear about the goals of using network approaches, whether they serve a purely descriptive goal or are explicitly understood as dependent and independent variables embedded in effect mechanism (Thatcher, 1998, pp. 410-411).

The scope and terms in the PAF have already been presented and distinguished from other similar network definitions in this subchapter.

Essentially, the literature on policy networks emphasizes that policy actors in policy networks always share one or more characteristics that serve as defining features of that network. Sometimes these characteristics are rather loose, such as repeated engagement with and reflection on a particular policy issue. Sometimes the defining characteristics of a policy network are narrower and include only those who share similar beliefs (such as advocacy coalitions). In the view of other perspectives, networks are mere products of institutional settings and follow the rules and scope that are institutionally imposed on them for rational cost-reducing interests, as is the perspective of the Actor-Centered Institutionalism (Bevir & Richards, 2009, p. 6; Scharpf, 1997).

Complementing these perspectives, the PAF brings a new approach to research on network formation in policy process research. The first aspect is the role of shared biographies in creating a sense of belonging and thus the roots for cooperation. Second, social psychological insights into the dynamics of group processes have only partially found their way into these studies. Among the rare contributions are those dealing with learning processes across advocacy coalitions (Koebele, 2019; Wagner & Ylä-Anttila, 2020, p. 196) or biased perception in the context of devil and angel shifts (Nilsson et al., 2020). The main argument made in the following chapters is that a focus on these group-based drivers of identification with a policy program can explain major policy change beyond existing policy network approaches. The main goal of the empirical analysis is to systematically test hypotheses about which institutional influences promote programmatic action and the success of programmatic groups.

References

Ackermann, K. (2016). Individual Differences and Political Contexts – The Role of Personality Traits and Direct Democracy in Explaining Political Protest. *Swiss Political Science Review, 23*(1), 21–49. https://doi.org/10.1111/spsr.12227

Ackrill, R., Kay, A., & Zahariadis, N. (2013). Ambiguity, Multiple Streams, and EU Policy. *Journal of European Public Policy, 20*(6), 871–887. https://doi.org/10.1080/13501763.2013.781824

Adler, E. (1992). The Emergence of Cooperation: National Epistemic Communities and the International Evolution of the Idea of Nuclear Arms Control. *International Organization, 46*(1), 101–145. Retrieved from www.jstor.org/stable/2706953

Adler, E., & Haas, P. M. (1992). Conclusion: Epistemic Communities, World Order, and the Creation of a Reflective Research Program. *International Organization, 46*(1), 367–390. https://doi.org/10.1017/S0020818300001533

Ajzen, I. (1991). The Theory of Planned Behavior. *Organizational Behavior and Human Decision Processes, 50*(2), 179–211. https://doi.org/10.1016/0749-5978(91)90020-T

Ajzen, I., & Fishbein, M. (1980). *Understanding Attitudes and Predicting Social Behaviour.* Prentice-Hall.

Albright, E. A. (2011). Policy Change and Learning in Response to Extreme Flood Events in Hungary: An Advocacy Coalition Approach. *Policy Studies Journal, 39*(3), 485–511. https://doi.org/10.1111/j.1541-0072.2011.00418.x

Ardıç, Ö., Annema, J. A., & Wee, B. V. (2015). Non-implementation of Road Pricing Policy in the Netherlands: An Application of the 'Advocacy Coalition Framework'. *European Journal of Transport and Infrastructure Research, 15*(2), 116–146. https://doi.org/10.18757/ejtir.2015.15.2.3065

Aschhoff, N., & Vogel, R. (2019). Something Old, Something New, Something Borrowed: Explaining Varieties of Professionalism in Citizen Collaboration Through Identity Theory. *Public Administration, 1*, 1. https://doi.org/10.1111/padm.12589

Atkinson, M. M., & Coleman, W. D. (1992). Policy Networks, Policy Communities and the Problems of Governance. *Governance, 5*(2), 154–180. https://doi.org/10.1111/j.1468-0491.1992.tb00034.x

Atkinson, R., Held, G., & Jeffares, S. (2011). Theories of Discourse and Narrative: What Do They Mean for Governance and Policy? In R. Atkinson, G. Terizakis, & K. Zimmermann (Eds.), *Sustainability in European Environmental Policy. Challenges of Governance and Knowledge* (pp. 115–130). Routledge.

Bachner, J., & Hill, K. W. (2014). Advances in Public Opinion and Policy Attitudes Research. *Policy Studies Journal, 42*(S1), S51–S70. https://doi.org/10.1111/psj.12052

Bäck, H., Renström, E. A., & Sivén, D. (2020). The Social Network: How Friends' Online Behavior and Belongingness Needs Influence Political Activity. *Policy & Internet, n/a*(n/a). doi:https://doi.org/10.1002/poi3.240

Bakir, C., & Jarvis, D. S. L. (2017). Contextualising the Context in Policy Entrepreneurship and Institutional Change. *Policy and Society, 36*(4), 465–478. https://doi.org/10.1080/14494035.2017.1393589

Bandelow, N. C., Hornung, J., & Smyrl, M. (2021). Theoretical Foundations of the Programmatic Action Framework (PAF). *European Policy Analysis, 7*(1), 14–27. https://doi.org/10.1002/epa2.1083

Bandelow, N. C., & Vogeler, C. S. (2019). Koalitionsverhandlungen als Entscheidungsfenster im deutschen politischen System? In R. Zohlnhöfer & T. Saalfeld (Eds.), *Zwischen Stillstand, Politikwandel und Krisenmanagement: Eine Bilanz der Regierung Merkel 2013-2017* (pp. 533–548). Springer Fachmedien Wiesbaden.

Bankert, A., Huddy, L., & Rosema, M. (2016). Measuring Partisanship as a Social Identity in Multi-Party Systems. *Political Behavior, 39*(1), 103–132. https://doi.org/10.1007/s11109-016-9349-5

Bartle, J., & Bellucci, P. (2009). *Political Parties and Partisanship: Social Identity and Individual Attitudes.* Routledge.

Baumgartner, F. R., Jones, B. D., & Mortensen, P. B. (2017). Punctuated Equilibrium Theory: Explaining Stability and Change in Public Policymaking. In C. M. Weible & P. A. Sabatier (Eds.), *Theories of the Policy Process* (4th ed., pp. 55–102). Westview Press.

Béland, D. (2016). Kingdon Reconsidered: Ideas, Interests and Institutions in Comparative Policy Analysis. *Journal of Comparative Policy Analysis: Research and Practice, 18*(3), 228–242. https://doi.org/10.1080/1387698 8.2015.1029770

Béland, D. (2019). *How Ideas and Institutions Shape the Politics of Public Policy* doi:https://doi.org/10.1017/9781108634700

Béland, D., & Howlett, M. (2016). The Role and Impact of the Multiple-Streams Approach in Comparative Policy Analysis. *Journal of Comparative Policy Analysis: Research and Practice, 18*(3), 221–227. https://doi.org/10.108 0/13876988.2016.1174410

Béland, D., Howlett, M., & Mukherjee, I. (2018). Instrument Constituencies and Public Policy-making: An Introduction. *Policy and Society, 37*(1), 1–13. https://doi.org/10.1080/14494035.2017.1375249

Berardo, R. (2008). Generalized Trust in Multi-organizational Policy Arenas: Studying Its Emergence from a Network Perspective. *Political Research Quarterly, 62*(1), 178–189. https://doi.org/10.1177/1065912907312982

Bevir, M., & Richards, D. (2009). Decentring Policy Networks: A Theoretical Agenda. *Public Administration, 87*(1), 3–14. https://doi.org/10.1111/j.1467-9299.2008.01736.x

Bhanot, S. P., & Linos, E. (2019). Behavioral Public Administration: Past, Present, and Future. *Public Administration Review, n/a*(n/a). doi:https://doi.org/10.1111/puar.13129

Birkland, T. A. (1998). Focusing Events, Mobilization, and Agenda Setting. *Journal of Public Policy, 18*(1), 53–74. https://doi.org/10.1017/S0143814X98000038

Blum, S. (2017). The Multiple-Streams Framework and Knowledge Utilization. Argumentative Couplings of Problem, Policy, and Politics Issues. *European Policy Analysis, 4*(1), 94–117. https://doi.org/10.1002/epa2.1029

Brandt, M. J., Sibley, C. G., & Osborne, D. (2019). What Is Central to Political Belief System Networks? *Personality and Social Psychology Bulletin, 45*(9), 1352–1364. https://doi.org/10.1177/0146167218824354

Brewer, M. B. (1991). The Social Self: On Being the Same and Different at the Same Time. *Personality and Social Psychology Bulletin, 17*(5), 475–482. https://doi.org/10.1177/0146167291175001

Bromley-Trujillo, R., & Poe, J. (2020). The Importance of Salience: Public Opinion and State Policy Action on Climate Change. *Journal of Public Policy, 40*(2), 280–304. https://doi.org/10.1017/S0143814X18000375

Brunner, S. (2008). Understanding Policy Change: Multiple Streams and Emissions Trading in Germany. *Global Environmental Change, 18*(3), 501–507. https://doi.org/10.1016/j.gloenvcha.2008.05.003

Bulkeley, H. (2000). Discourse Coalitions and the Australian Climate Change Policy Network. *Environment and Planning C: Government and Policy, 18*(6), 727–748. https://doi.org/10.1068/c9905j

Cairney, P. (2018). Three Habits of Successful Policy Entrepreneurs. *Policy & Politics, 46*(2), 199–215. https://doi.org/10.1332/030557 318x15230056771696

Calanni, J. C., Siddiki, S. N., Weible, C. M., & Leach, W. D. (2014). Explaining Coordination in Collaborative Partnerships and Clarifying the Scope of the Belief Homophily Hypothesis. *Journal of Public Administration Research and Theory, 25*(3), 901–927. https://doi.org/10.1093/jopart/mut080

Capano, G., & Lippi, A. (2017). How Policy Instruments Are Chosen: Patterns of Decision Makers' Choices. *Policy Sciences, 50*(2), 269–293. https://doi.org/10.1007/s11077-016-9267-8

Carlsson, L. (2000). Policy Networks as Collective Action. *Policy Studies Journal, 28*(3), 502–520. https://doi.org/10.1111/j.1541-0072.2000.tb02045.x

Carstensen, M. B. (2011). Paradigm Man vs. the Bricoleur: Bricolage as an Alternative Vision of Agency in Ideational Change. *European Political Science Review, 3*(1), 147–167. https://doi.org/10.1017/S1755773910000342

Cohen, M. D., March, J. G., & Olsen, J. P. (1972). A Garbage Can Model of Organizational Choice. *Administrative Science Quarterly, 17*(1), 1–25. https://doi.org/10.2307/2392088

Converse, P. E. (2006). The Nature of Belief Systems in Mass Publics (1964). *Critical Review, 18*(1-3), 1–74. https://doi.org/10.1080/08913810608443650

Crow, D. A., Albright, E. A., Ely, T., Koebele, E., & Lawhon, L. (2018). Do Disasters Lead to Learning? Financial Policy Change in Local Government. *Review of Policy Research, 35*(4), 564–589. https://doi.org/10.1111/ropr.12297

Daigneault, P.-M. (2014). Reassessing the Concept of Policy Paradigm: Aligning Ontology and Methodology in Policy Studies. *Journal of European Public Policy, 21*(3), 453–469. https://doi.org/10.1080/13501763.2013.834071

DeLeon, P., & Varda, D. M. (2009). Toward a Theory of Collaborative Policy Networks: Identifying Structural Tendencies. *Policy Studies Journal, 37*(1), 59–74. https://doi.org/10.1111/j.1541-0072.2008.00295.x

Deruelle, T. (2016). Bricolage or Entrepreneurship?: Lessons from the Creation of the European Centre for Disease Prevention and Control. *European Policy Analysis, 2*(2), 43–67. https://doi.org/10.18278/epa.2.2.4

Devine-Wright, P., & Howes, Y. (2010). Disruption to Place Attachment and the Protection of Restorative Environments: A Wind Energy Case Study. *Journal of Environmental Psychology, 30*(3), 271–280. https://doi.org/10.1016/j. jenvp.2010.01.008

Dinesen, P. T., Nørgaard, A. S., & Klemmensen, R. (2014). The Civic Personality: Personality and Democratic Citizenship. *Political Studies, 62*(S1), 134–152. https://doi.org/10.1111/1467-9248.12094

Duckitt, J., & Sibley, C. G. (2016). Personality, Ideological Attitudes, and Group Identity as Predictors of Political Behavior in Majority and Minority Ethnic Groups. *Political Psychology, 37*(1), 109–124. https://doi.org/10.1111/ pops.12222

Dudley, G., & Richardson, J. (1996). Why Does Policy Change Over Time? Adversarial Policy Communities, Alternative Policy Arenas, and British Trunk Roads Policy 1945–95. *Journal of European Public Policy, 3*(1), 63–83. https:// doi.org/10.1080/13501769608407018

Duina, F. (2019). Why the Excitement? Values, Identities, and the Politicization of EU Trade Policy with North America. *Journal of European Public Policy, 1*, 1–17. https://doi.org/10.1080/13501763.2019.1678056

Dunlop, C. A., & Radaelli, C. M. (2017). Learning in the Bath-Tub: The Micro and Macro Dimensions of the Causal Relationship between Learning and Policy Change. *Policy and Society, 36*(2), 304–319. https://doi.org/10.108 0/14494035.2017.1321232

Dunlop, C. A., & Radaelli, C. M. (2018). Does Policy Learning Meet the Standards of an Analytical Framework of the Policy Process? *Policy Studies Journal.* https://doi.org/10.1111/psj.12250

Durr, R. H. (1993). What Moves Policy Sentiment? *American Political Science Review, 87*(1), 158–170. https://doi.org/10.2307/2938963

Egan, P. J. (2019). Identity as Dependent Variable: How Americans Shift Their Identities to Align with Their Politics. *American Journal of Political Science, n/a*(n/a). doi:https://doi.org/10.1111/ajps.12496

Enns, P. K., & Kellstedt, P. M. (2008). Policy Mood and Political Sophistication: Why Everybody Moves Mood. *British Journal of Political Science, 38*(3), 433–454. https://doi.org/10.1017/S0007123408000227

Eriksson, L. (2017). The Role of Organizational Identities for Policy Integration Processes – Managing Sustainable Transport Development. *Public Organization Review, 17*(4), 525–544. https://doi.org/10.1007/s11115-016-0348-0

Ewert, B. (2019). Moving Beyond the Obsession with Nudging Individual Behaviour: Towards a Broader Understanding of Behavioural Public Policy. *Public Policy and Administration, 0952076719889090.* https://doi.org/ 10.1177/0952076719889090

Fenger, M., & Klok, P.-J. (2001). Interdependency, Beliefs, and Coalition Behavior: A Contribution to the Advocacy Coalition Framework. *Policy Sciences, 34*(2), 157–170. https://doi.org/10.1023/A:1010330511419

Fischer, M. (2015). Institutions and Coalitions in Policy Processes: A Cross-sectoral Comparison. *Journal of Public Policy, 35*(2), 245–268. https://doi.org/10.1017/S0143814X14000166

Fischer, M., Ingold, K., Sciarini, P., & Varone, F. (2016). Dealing With Bad Guys: Actor- and Process-level Determinants of the "Devil Shift" in Policy Making. *Journal of Public Policy, 36*(2), 309–334. https://doi.org/10.1017/S0143814X15000021

Fischer, M., & Sciarini, P. (2015). Drivers of Collaboration in Political Decision Making: A Cross-Sector Perspective. *The Journal of Politics, 78*(1), 63–74. https://doi.org/10.1086/683061

Fisher, P. (2020). Generational Replacement and the Impending Transformation of the American Electorate. *Politics & Policy, 48*(1), 38–68. https://doi.org/10.1111/polp.12340

Forester, J. (1984). Bounded Rationality and the Politics of Muddling Through. *Public Administration Review, 44*(1), 23.

Fowler, L. (2018). Problems, Politics, and Policy Streams in Policy Implementation. *Governance, 0*, 1. https://doi.org/10.1111/gove.12382

Fowler, L. (2020). Using the Multiple Streams Framework to Connect Policy Adoption to Implementation. *Policy Studies Journal, n/a*(n/a). doi:https://doi.org/10.1111/psj.12381

Francesco, F. D., & Guaschino, E. (2020). Reframing Knowledge: A Comparison of OECD and World Bank Discourse on Public Governance Reform. *Policy and Society, 39*(1), 113–128. https://doi.org/10.1080/14494035.2019.1609391

Freeman, J. L., & Stevens, J. P. (1987). A Theoretical and Conceptual Reexamination of Subsystem Politics. *Public Policy and Administration, 2*(1), 9–24. https://doi.org/10.1177/095207678700200102

Freitag, M., & Bauer, P. C. (2016). Personality Traits and the Propensity to Trust Friends and Strangers. *The Social Science Journal, 53*(4), 467–476. https://doi.org/10.1016/j.soscij.2015.12.002

Genieys, W. (2010). *The New Custodians of the State: Programmatic Elites in French Society*. Transaction Publishers.

Genieys, W., & Hassenteufel, P. (2001). Entre les politiques publiques et la politique: l'émergence d'une "élite du Welfare"? *Revue française des affaires sociales, 4*(4), 41–50.

Genieys, W., & Hassenteufel, P. (2012). Comprendre le changement dans les politiques publiques ? L'approche programmatique. Retrieved from https://hal.archives-ouvertes.fr/hal-01401805

Genieys, W., & Michel, L. (2005). The Invention of the Leclerc Tank: The Singular Role of a Project Elite. *French Politics, 3*(3), 187–210. https://doi.org/10.1057/palgrave.fp.8200086

Genieys, W., & Smyrl, M. (2008a). Competing Elites, Legitimate Authority, Structured Ideas. In W. Genieys & M. Smyrl (Eds.), *Elites, Ideas, and the Evolution of Public Policy* (pp. 19–51). Palgrave Macmillan.

Genieys, W., & Smyrl, M. (2008b). *Elites, Ideas, and the Evolution of Public Policy* (1st ed.). Palgrave Macmillan.

Genieys, W., & Smyrl, M. (2008c). Inside the Autonomous State: Programmatic Elites in the Reform of French Health Policy. *Governance, 21*(1), 75–93. https://doi.org/10.1111/j.1468-0491.2007.00386.x

Gerber, A. S., Green, D. P., & Larimer, C. W. (2008). Social Pressure and Voter Turnout: Evidence from a Large-Scale Field Experiment. *American Political Science Review, 102*(1), 33–48. https://doi.org/10.1017/S000305540808009X

Goldberg, L. R. (1990). An Alternative "Description of Personality": The Big-Five Factor Structure. *Journal of Personality and Social Psychology, 59*(6), 1216–1229. https://doi.org/10.1037/0022-3514.59.6.1216

Goren, P. (2005). Party Identification and Core Political Values. *American Journal of Political Science, 49*(4), 881–896.

Gosling, S. D., Rentfrow, P. J., & Swann, W. B. (2003). A Very Brief Measure of the Big-Five Personality Domains. *Journal of Research in Personality, 37*(6), 504–528. https://doi.org/10.1016/S0092-6566(03)00046-1

Grant, W., & MacNamara, A. (1995). When Policy Communities Intersect: The Case of Agriculture and Banking. *Political Studies, 43*(3), 509–515. https://doi.org/10.1111/j.1467-9248.1995.tb00319.x

Greene, S. (1999). Understanding Party Identification: A Social Identity Approach. *Political Psychology, 20*(2), 393–403. https://doi.org/10.1111/0162-895X.00150

Greene, S. (2004). Social Identity Theory and Party Identification*. *Social Science Quarterly, 85*(1), 136–153. https://doi.org/10.1111/j.0038-4941.2004.08501010.x

Grimmelikhuijsen, S., Jilke, S., Olsen, A. L., & Tummers, L. (2017). Behavioral Public Administration: Combining Insights from Public Administration and Psychology. *Public Administration Review, 77*(1), 45–56. https://doi.org/10.1111/puar.12609

Grødem, A. S., & Hippe, J. M. (2019). The Expertise of Politicians and Their Role in Epistemic Communities. *Policy & Politics, 47*, 561–577.

Gronow, A., Ylä-Anttila, T., Carson, M., & Edling, C. (2019). Divergent Neighbors: Corporatism and Climate Policy Networks in Finland and Sweden. *Environmental Politics, 28*(6), 1061–1083. https://doi.org/10.1080/09644016.2019.1625149

Gupta, K. (2014). A Comparative Policy Analysis of Coalition Strategies: Case Studies of Nuclear Energy and Forest Management in India. *Journal of Comparative Policy Analysis: Research and Practice, 16*(4), 356–372. https://doi.org/10.1080/13876988.2014.886812

Gupta, K., Ripberger, J., & Wehde, W. (2018). Advocacy Group Messaging on Social Media: Using the Narrative Policy Framework to Study Twitter Messages about Nuclear Energy Policy in the United States. *Policy Studies Journal, 46*(1), 119–136. https://doi.org/10.1111/psj.12176

Haas, P. M. (1992). Introduction: Epistemic Communities and International Policy Coordination. *International Organization, 46*(1), 1–35.

Haelg, L., Sewerin, S., & Schmidt, T. S. (2020). The Role of Actors in the Policy Design Process: Introducing Design Coalitions to Explain Policy Output. *Policy Sciences, 53*(2), 309–347. https://doi.org/10.1007/s11077-019-09365-z

Hall, P. A. (1993). Policy Paradigms, Social Learning, and the State: The Case of Economic Policymaking in Britain. *Comparative Politics, 25*(3), 275–296. https://doi.org/10.2307/422246

Hann, A. (1995). Sharpening up Sabatier: Belief Systems and Public Policy. *Politics, 15*(1), 19–26. https://doi.org/10.1111/j.1467-9256.1995.tb00016.x

Hassenteufel, P., & Genieys, W. (2021). The Programmatic Action Framework: An Empirical Assessment. *European Policy Analysis, 7*(1), 28–47. https://doi.org/10.1002/epa2.1088

Hassenteufel, P., Smyrl, M., Genieys, W., & Moreno-Fuentes, F. J. (2010). Programmatic Actors and the Transformation of European Health Care States. *Journal of Health Politics, Policy and Law, 35*(4), 517–538. https://doi.org/1 0.1215/03616878-2010-015

Heaney, M. T. (2004). Issue Networks, Information, and Interest Group Alliances: The Case of Wisconsin Welfare Politics, 1993–99. *State Politics & Policy Quarterly, 4*(3), 237–270. https://doi.org/10.1177/153244000400400301

Heclo, H. (1978). Issue Networks and the Executive Establishment. In A. King (Ed.), *The New American Political System* (pp. 413–422). American Enterprise Institute.

Heikkila, T., Berardo, R., Weible, C. M., & Yi, H. (2019). A Comparative View of Advocacy Coalitions: Exploring Shale Development Politics in the United States, Argentina, and China. *Journal of Comparative Policy Analysis: Research and Practice, 21*(2), 151–166. https://doi.org/10.1080/1387698 8.2017.1405551

Henry, A. D. (2011a). Belief-Oriented Segregation in Policy Networks. *Procedia - Social and Behavioral Sciences, 22,* 14–25. https://doi.org/10.1016/j. sbspro.2011.07.052

Henry, A. D. (2011b). Ideology, Power, and the Structure of Policy Networks. *Policy Studies Journal, 39*(3), 361–383. https://doi.org/10.1111/j.1541-0072.2011.00413.x

Herweg, N. (2016). Explaining European Agenda-setting Using the Multiple Streams Framework: the Case of European Natural Gas Regulation. *Policy Sciences, 49*(1), 13–33. https://doi.org/10.1007/s11077-015-9231-z

Herweg, N., Huß, C., & Zohlnhöfer, R. (2015). Straightening the Three Streams: Theorizing Extensions of the Multiple Streams Framework. *European Journal of Political Research, 54*(3), 435–449.

Herweg, N., Zahariadis, N., & Zohlnhöfer, R. (2017). The Multiple Streams Framework: Foundations, Refinements, and Empirical Applications. In C. M. Weible & P. A. Sabatier (Eds.), *Theories of the Policy Process* (4th ed., pp. 17–53). Westview Press.

Hildebrandt, A., & Trüdinger, E.-M. (2020). History is not Bunk. Tradition, Political Economy and Regional Identity in the German Länder. *German Politics, 1*, 1–18. https://doi.org/10.1080/09644008.2020.1749265

Hogg, M. A., Abrams, D., & Brewer, M. B. (2017). Social Identity: The Role of Self in Group Processes and Intergroup Relations. *Group Processes & Intergroup Relations, 20*(5), 570–581. https://doi.org/10.1177/1368430217690909

Hogg, M. A., Terry, D. J., & White, K. M. (1995). A Tale of Two Theories: A Critical Comparison of Identity Theory with Social Identity Theory. *Social Psychology Quarterly, 58*(4), 255–269. https://doi.org/10.2307/2787127

Hornsey, M. J. (2008). Social Identity Theory and Self-Categorization Theory: A Historical Review. *Social and Personality Psychology Compass, 2*(1), 204–222. https://doi.org/10.1111/j.1751-9004.2007.00066.x

Hornung, J., & Bandelow, N. C. (2020). The Programmatic Elite in German Health Policy: Collective Action and Sectoral History. *Public Policy and Administration, 35*(3), 247–265. https://doi.org/10.1177/0952076718798887

Hornung, J., Bandelow, N. C., & Vogeler, C. S. (2019). Social Identities in the Policy Process. *Policy Sciences, 52*(2), 211–231. https://doi.org/10.1007/s11077-018-9340-6

Howlett, M. (2018). Moving Policy Implementation Theory Forward: A Multiple Streams/Critical Juncture Approach. *Public Policy and Administration, 34*(4), 405–430. https://doi.org/10.1177/0952076718775791

Howlett, M., Capano, G., & Ramesh, M. (2018). Designing for Robustness: Surprise, Agility and Improvisation in Policy Design. *Policy and Society, 37*(4), 405–421. https://doi.org/10.1080/14494035.2018.1504488

Howlett, M., Kim, J., & Weaver, P. (2006). Assessing Instrument Mixes through Program- and Agency-Level Data: Methodological Issues in Contemporary Implementation Research. *Review of Policy Research, 23*(1), 129–151. https://doi.org/10.1111/j.1541-1338.2006.00189.x

Howlett, M., & Ramesh, M. (1998). Policy Subsystem Configurations and Policy Change: Operationalizing the Postpositivist Analysis of the Politics of the Policy process. *Policy Studies Journal, 26*(3), 466–481. https://doi.org/10.1111/j.1541-0072.1998.tb01913.x

Huddy, L. (2001). From Social to Political Identity: A Critical Examination of Social Identity Theory. *Political Psychology, 22*(1), 127–156. https://doi.org/10.1111/0162-895X.00230

Huddy, L., Mason, L., & Aarøe, L. (2015). Expressive Partisanship: Campaign Involvement, Political Emotion, and Partisan Identity. *American Political Science Review, 109*(1), 1–17. https://doi.org/10.1017/S0003055414000604

Ingold, K. (2011). Network Structures within Policy Processes: Coalitions, Power, and Brokerage in Swiss Climate Policy. *Policy Studies Journal, 39*(3), 435–459. https://doi.org/10.1111/j.1541-0072.2011.00416.x

Ingold, K., & Leifeld, P. (2014). Structural and Institutional Determinants of Influence Reputation: A Comparison of Collaborative and Adversarial Policy Networks in Decision Making and Implementation. *Journal of Public Administration Research and Theory, 26*(1), 1–18. https://doi.org/10.1093/jopart/muu043

Ingram, M., Ingram, H., & Lejano, R. (2019). Environmental Action in the Anthropocene: The Power of Narrative-Networks. *Journal of Environmental Policy & Planning, 21*(5), 492–503. https://doi.org/10.1080/1523908X.2015.1113513

Iyengar, S., & Westwood, S. J. (2015). Fear and Loathing across Party Lines: New Evidence on Group Polarization. *American Journal of Political Science, 59*(3), 690–707. https://doi.org/10.1111/ajps.12152

Jenkins-Smith, H. C., Nohrstedt, D., Weible, C. M., & Ingold, K. (2017). The Advocacy Coalition Framework: An Overview of the Research Program. In C. M. Weible & P. A. Sabatier (Eds.), *Theories of the Policy Process* (pp. 135–170). Westview Press.

Jenkins-Smith, H. C., Silva, C. L., Gupta, K., & Ripberger, J. T. (2014). Belief System Continuity and Change in Policy Advocacy Coalitions: Using Cultural Theory to Specify Belief Systems, Coalitions, and Sources of Change. *Policy Studies Journal, 42*(4), 484–508. https://doi.org/10.1111/psj.12071

Johannesson, L., & Qvist, M. (2020). Navigating the Policy Stream: Contested Solutions and Organizational Strategies of Policy Entrepreneurship. *International Review of Public Policy, 2*(1), 1–21.

John, P., & Stoker, G. (2019). Rethinking the Role of Experts and Expertise in Behavioural Public Policy. *Policy & Politics, 47*(2), 209–226.

Jones, B. D. (1999). Bounded Rationality. *Annual Review of Political Science, 2*, 291–321.

Jones, M. D. (2011). Leading the Way to Compromise? Cultural Theory and Climate Change Opinion. *PS. Political Science & Politics, 44*(4), 720–725. https://doi.org/10.1017/S104909651100134X

Jones, M. D., Peterson, H. L., Pierce, J. J., Herweg, N., Bernal, A., Lamberta Raney, H., & Zahariadis, N. (2016). A River Runs Through It: A Multiple Streams Meta-Review. *Policy Studies Journal, 44*(1), 13–36. https://doi.org/10.1111/psj.12115

Jordan, A. G. (1981). Iron Triangles, Woolly Corporatism and Elastic Nets: Images of the Policy Process. *Journal of Public Policy, 1*(1), 95–123. https://doi.org/10.1017/S0143814X00001379

Jordan, G. (1990). Sub-Governments, Policy Communities and Networks: Refilling the Old Bottles? *Journal of Theoretical Politics, 2*(3), 319–338. https://doi.org/10.1177/0951692890002003004

Jordan, G., & Maloney, W. A. (1997). Accounting for Sub Governments: Explaining the Persistence of Policy Communities. *Administration & Society, 29*(5), 557–583. https://doi.org/10.1177/009539979702900503

Jordan, G., & Schubert, K. (1992). A Preliminary Ordering of Policy Network Labels. *European Journal of Political Research, 21*(1-2), 7–27. https://doi.org/10.1111/j.1475-6765.1992.tb00286.x

Kagan, J. A. (2019). Multiple Streams in Hawaii: How the Aloha State Adopted a 100% Renewable Portfolio Standard. *Review of Policy Research, 36*(2), 217–241. https://doi.org/10.1111/ropr.12323

Kalafatis, S. E., Lemos, M. C., Lo, Y.-J., & Frank, K. A. (2015). Increasing Information Usability for Climate Adaptation: The Role of Knowledge Networks and Communities of Practice. *Global Environmental Change, 32*, 30–39. https://doi.org/10.1016/j.gloenvcha.2015.02.007

Keating, M., Cairney, P., & Hepburn, E. (2009). Territorial Policy Communities and Devolution in the UK. *Cambridge Journal of Regions, Economy and Society, 2*(1), 51–66. https://doi.org/10.1093/cjres/rsn024

Keeler, J. T. S. (1993). Executive Power and Policy-making Patterns in France: Gauging the Impact of Fifth Republic Institutions. *West European Politics, 16*(4), 518–544. https://doi.org/10.1080/01402389308424989

Ki, N., Kwak, C.-G., & Song, M. (2020). Strength of Strong Ties in Intercity Government Information Sharing and County Jurisdictional Boundaries. *Public Administration Review, 80*(1), 23–35. https://doi.org/10.1111/puar.13135

Kingdon, J. W. (2003). *Agendas, Alternatives, and Public Policies* (2nd ed.). Pearson Education.

Kirst, M. W., Meister, G., & Rowley, S. R. (1984). Policy Issue Networks: Their Influence on State Policymaking. *Policy Studies Journal, 13*(2), 247–263. https://doi.org/10.1111/j.1541-0072.1984.tb00338.x

Knaggård, Å. (2015). The Multiple Streams Framework and the Problem Broker. *European Journal of Political Research, 54*(3), 450–465. https://doi.org/10.1111/1475-6765.12097

Knoke, D., & Kostiuchenko, T. (2017). Power Structures of Policy Networks. In J. N. Victor, A. H. Montgomery, M. Lubell, D. Knoke, & T. Kostiuchenko (Eds.), *The Oxford Handbook of Political Networks*. Oxford University Press.

Koebele, E. A. (2018). Integrating Collaborative Governance Theory with the Advocacy Coalition Framework. *Journal of Public Policy, 1-30*, 1. https://doi.org/10.1017/s0143814x18000041

Koebele, E. A. (2019). Cross-Coalition Coordination in Collaborative Environmental Governance Processes. *Policy Studies Journal, 0*, 1. https://doi.org/10.1111/psj.12306

Kübler, D. (2001). Understanding Policy Change with the Advocacy Coalition Framework: An Application to Swiss Drug Policy. *Journal of European Public Policy, 8*(4), 623–641. https://doi.org/10.1080/13501760110064429

Kuhn, T., & Nicoli, F. (2020). Collective Identities and the Integration of Core State Powers: Introduction to the Special Issue. *JCMS: Journal of Common Market Studies, 58*(1), 3–20. https://doi.org/10.1111/jcms.12985

Lakatos, I., & Musgrave, A. (1970). *Criticism and the Growth of Knowledge.* University Press.

Laumann, E. O., & Knoke, D. (1987). *The Organizational State: Social Choice in National Policy Domains.* University of Wisconsin Press.

Laumann, E. O., Knoke, D., & Kim, Y.-H. (1985). An Organizational Approach to State Policy Formation: A Comparative Study of Energy and Health Domains. *American Sociological Review, 50*(1), 1–19. https://doi.org/10.2307/2095336

Lazer, D., Rubineau, B., Chetkovich, C., Katz, N., & Neblo, M. (2010). The Coevolution of Networks and Political Attitudes. *Political Communication, 27*(3), 248–274. https://doi.org/10.1080/10584609.2010.500187

Leach, W. D., & Sabatier, P. A. (2005). To Trust an Adversary: Integrating Rational and Psychological Models of Collaborative Policymaking. *American Political Science Review, 99*(4), 491–503. https://doi.org/10.1017/S000305540505183X

Lejano, R., Chui, E., Lam, T., & Wong, J. (2017). Collective Action as Narrativity and Praxis: Theory and Application to Hong Kong's Urban Protest Movements. *Public Policy and Administration, 33*(3), 260–289. https://doi.org/10.1177/0952076717699262

Leong, C., & Howlett, M. (2020). Theorizing the Behavioral State: Resolving the Theory-practice Paradox of Policy Sciences. *Public Policy and Administration, 0952076720977588.* https://doi.org/10.1177/0952076720977588

Lertzman, K., Rayner, J., & Wilson, J. (1996). Learning and Change in the British Columbia Forest Policy Sector: A Consideration of Sabatier's Advocacy Coalition Framework. *Canadian Journal of Political Science, 29*(1), 111–133. https://doi.org/10.1017/S0008423900007265

Lichtmannegger, C., & Tobias, B. (2020). The Interaction of Multiple Drivers of Intra-organizational Change in Ministerial Administrations: A Study of Three Decades of Structural Reforms in the Austrian Ministry of Agriculture. *Public Policy and Administration, 0952076720904439.* https://doi.org/10.1177/0952076720904439

Lindblom, C. E. (1959). The Science of "Muddling Through". *Public Administration Review, 19*(2), 79–88.

Lodge, M. (2019). How Far to Nudge? Assessing Behavioural Public Policy. *Public Administration, 0,* 1. https://doi.org/10.1111/padm.12582

Lubell, M. (2003). Collaborative Institutions, Belief-Systems, and Perceived Policy Effectiveness. *Political Research Quarterly, 56*(3), 309–323. https://doi.org/10.1177/106591290305600306

Lubell, M. (2007). Familiarity Breeds Trust: Collective Action in a Policy Domain. *Journal of Politics, 69*(1), 237–250. https://doi.org/10.1111/j.1468-2508.2007.00507.x

March, J. G. (1978). Bounded Rationality, Ambiguity, and the Engineering of Choice. *The Bell Journal of Economics, 9*(2), 587–608. https://doi.org/10.2307/3003600

Markard, J., Suter, M., & Ingold, K. (2016). Socio-technical Transitions and Policy Change – Advocacy Coalitions in Swiss Energy Policy. *Environmental Innovation and Societal Transitions, 18,* 215–237. https://doi.org/10.1016/j.eist.2015.05.003

McCool, D. (1998). The Subsystem Family of Concepts: A Critique and a Proposal. *Political Research Quarterly, 51*(2), 551–570. https://doi.org/10.1177/106591299805100213

McCrae, R. R., & Costa, P. T. (1987). Validation of the Five-factor Model of Personality Across Instruments and Observers. *Journal of Personality and Social Psychology, 52*(1), 81–90. https://doi.org/10.1037/0022-3514.52.1.81

McGee, Z. A., & Jones, B. D. (2019). Reconceptualizing the Policy Subsystem: Integration with Complexity Theory and Social Network Analysis. *Policy Studies Journal, 47*(S1), S138–S158. https://doi.org/10.1111/psj.12319

McPherson, M., Smith-Lovin, L., & Cook, J. M. (2001). Birds of a Feather: Homophily in Social Networks. *Annual Review of Sociology, 27*(1), 415–444. https://doi.org/10.1146/annurev.soc.27.1.415

Meijerink, S. (2005). Understanding Policy Stability and Change. The Interplay of Advocacy Coalitions and Epistemic Communities, Windows of Opportunity, and Dutch Coastal Flooding Policy 1945–2003. *Journal of European Public Policy, 12*(6), 1060–1077. https://doi.org/10.1080/13501760500270745

Metz, F., Lieberherr, E., Schmucki, A., & Huber, R. (2020). Policy Change Through Negotiated Agreements: The Case of Greening Swiss Agricultural Policy. *Policy Studies Journal, n/a*(n/a). doi:https://doi.org/10.1111/psj.12417

Michel, L. (2008). The French Cement Industry and the New Politics of the Environment. In W. Genieys & M. Smyrl (Eds.), *Elites, Ideas, and the Evolution of Public Policy* (pp. 152–167). Palgrave Macmillan.

Millar, H., Lesch, M., & White, L. A. (2019). Connecting Models of the Individual and Policy Change Processes: a Research Agenda. *Policy Sciences, 52*(1), 97–118. https://doi.org/10.1007/s11077-018-9327-3

Miller, H. T., & Demir, T. (2007). Policy Communities. In F. Fischer, G. J. Miller, & M. S. Sidney (Eds.), *Handbook of Public Policy Analysis. Theory, Politics, and Methods* (pp. 137–147). CRC Press.

Mills, C. W. (2000). *The Power Elite.* Oxford University Press.

Mintrom, M., & Norman, P. (2009). Policy Entrepreneurship and Policy Change. *Policy Studies Journal, 37*(4), 649–667. https://doi.org/10.1111/j.1541-0072.2009.00329.x

Moyson, S. (2017). Cognition and Policy Change: The Consistency of Policy Learning in the Advocacy Coalition Framework. *Policy and Society, 36*(2), 320–344. https://doi.org/10.1080/14494035.2017.1322259

Mukherjee, I., & Howlett, M. (2015). Who is a Stream? Epistemic Communities, Instrument Constituencies and Advocacy Coalitions in Multiple Streams Subsystems. *Lee Kuan Yew School of Public Policy Research Paper No., 15-18* (Available at SSRN: https://ssrn.com/abstract=2593626). doi:https://doi.org/10.2139/ssrn.2593626

Nilsson, J., Sandström, A., & Nohrstedt, D. (2020). Beliefs, Social Identity, and the View of Opponents in Swedish Carnivore Management Policy. *Policy Sciences.* doi:https://doi.org/10.1007/s11077-020-09380-5

Nohrstedt, D., Weible, C. M., Ingold, K., & Henry, A. D. (2020). Comparing Policy Processes: Insights and Lessons from the Advocacy Coalition Framework Research Program. In B. G. Peters & G. Fontaine (Eds.), *Handbook of Research Methods and Applications in Comparative Policy Analysis* (pp. 67–89). Edward Elgar Publishing Limited.

Nowlin, M. C. (2011). Theories of the Policy Process: State of the Research and Emerging Trends. *Policy Studies Journal, 39*(s1), 41–60. https://doi.org/10.1111/j.1541-0072.2010.00389_4.x

Nyland, J. (1995). Issue Networks and Nonprofit Organizations. *Review of Policy Research, 14*(1-2), 195–204. https://doi.org/10.1111/j.1541-1338.1995.tb00632.x

Obinger, H. (2012). Generationen und Politikwandel: Die demografische Ausdünnung der Kriegskohorten und die Transformation des Interventionsstaates. *dms - der moderne staat - Zeitschrift für Public Policy, Recht und Management, 5*(1), 169–192.

Olofsson, K. L., Katz, J., Costie, D. P., Heikkila, T., & Weible, C. M. (2018). A Dominant Coalition and Policy Change: An Analysis of Shale Oil and Gas Politics in India. *Journal of Environmental Policy & Planning, 20*(5), 645–660. https://doi.org/10.1080/1523908X.2018.1493984

Osei, A., & Malang, T. (2016). Party, Ethnicity, or Region? Determinants of Informal Political Exchange in the Parliament of Ghana. *Party Politics, 24*(4), 410–420. https://doi.org/10.1177/1354068816663038

Padgett, S. (1990). Policy Style and Issue Environment: The Electricity Supply Sector in West Germany. *Journal of Public Policy, 10*(2), 165–193. https://doi.org/10.1017/S0143814X00004803

Pannowitsch, S. (2009). Institutionalized Healthcare Reform in Germany? Error Correction or Political Strategy? *German Policy Studies, 5*(1), 141–168.

Parsons, B. M. (2015). The Social Identity Politics of Peer Networks. *American Politics Research, 43*(4), 680–707. https://doi.org/10.117 7/1532673x14546856

Parsons, B. M. (2020). The Effects of Risk, Beliefs, and Trust in Education Policy Networks: The Case of Autism and Special Education. *Policy Studies Journal, 48*(1), 38–63. https://doi.org/10.1111/psj.12246

Peters, B. G., Capano, G., Howlett, M., Mukherjee, I., Chou, M.-H., & Ravinet, P. (2018). *Designing for Policy Effectiveness: Defining and Understanding a Concept.* https://doi.org/10.1017/9781108555081

Pierce, J. J., Peterson, H. L., & Hicks, K. C. (2020). Policy Change: An Advocacy Coalition Framework Perspective. *Policy Studies Journal, 48*(1), 64–86. https://doi.org/10.1111/psj.12223

Pierce, J. J., Peterson, H. L., Jones, M. D., Garrard, S. P., & Vu, T. (2017). There and Back Again: A Tale of the Advocacy Coalition Framework. *Policy Studies Journal, 45*(1), 13–46. https://doi.org/10.1111/psj.12197

Putnam, R. D. (1995). Bowling Alone: America's Declining Social Capital. *Journal of Democracy, 6*(1), 65–78.

Rahman Khan, S. (2012). The Sociology of Elites. *Annual Review of Sociology, 38*(1), 361–377. https://doi.org/10.1146/annurev-soc-071811-145542

Reardon, L. (2018). Networks and Problem Recognition: Advancing the Multiple Streams Approach. *Policy Sciences, 51*(4), 457–476. https://doi.org/10.1007/s11077-018-9330-8

Ren, Y., Harper, F. M., Drenner, S., Terveen, L., Kiesler, S., Riedl, J., & Kraut, R. E. (2012). Building Member Attachment in Online Communities: Applying Theories of Group Identity and Interpersonal Bonds. *MIS Quarterly, 36*(3), 841–864. https://doi.org/10.2307/41703483

Rhodes, R. A. W. (1990). Policy Networks: A British Perspective. *Journal of Theoretical Politics, 2*(3), 293–317. https://doi.org/10.1177/0951692890002003003

Rhodes, R. A. W. (2008). Policy Network Analysis. In M. Moran, M. Rein, & R. E. Goodin (Eds.), *The Oxford Handbook of Public Policy* (pp. 425–447). Oxford University Press.

Ripberger, J. T., Gupta, K., Silva, C. L., & Jenkins-Smith, H. C. (2014). Cultural Theory and the Measurement of Deep Core Beliefs Within the Advocacy Coalition Framework. *Policy Studies Journal, 42*(4), 509–527. https://doi.org/10.1111/psj.12074

Rouban, L. (1989). The Civil Service and the Policy of Administrative Modernization in France. *International Review of Administrative Sciences, 55*(3), 445–465. https://doi.org/10.1177/002085238905500306

Sabatier, P. A. (1987). Knowledge, Policy-Oriented Learning, and Policy Change: An Advocacy Coalition Framework. *Knowledge, 8*(4), 649–692. https://doi.org/10.1177/0164025987008004005

Sabatier, P. A. (1988). An Advocacy Coalition Framework of Policy Change and the Role of Policy-Oriented Learning Therein. *Policy Sciences, 21*(2-3), 129–168.

Sabatier, P. A., & Brasher, A. M. (1993). From Vague Consensus to Clearly Differentiated Coalitions: Environmental Policy at Lake Tahoe. In H. C. Jenkins-Smith (Ed.), *Policy Change and Learning: An Advocacy Coalition Approach* (pp. 177–208). Westview Press.

Sabatier, P. A., & Hunter, S. (1989). The Incorporation of Causal Perceptions into Models of Elite Belief Systems. *Western Political Quarterly, 42*(3), 229–261. https://doi.org/10.1177/106591298904200304

Sabatier, P. A., & Jenkins-Smith, H. C. (Eds.). (1993). *Policy Change and Learning: An Advocacy Coalition Approach.* Westview Press.

Sabatier, P. A., & Weible, C. M. (2007). The Advocacy Coalition Framework: Innovations and Clarifications. In P. A. Sabatier (Ed.), *Theories of the Policy Process* (pp. 189–220). Westview Press.

Sætren, H. (2016). Lost in Translation: Re-conceptualising the Multiple-Streams Framework Back to its Source of Inspiration. In R. Zohlnhöfer & F. W. Rüb (Eds.), *Decision-Making under Ambiguity and Time Constraints. Assessing the Multiple-Streams Framework* (pp. 21–33). ECPR Press.

Sandström, A., & Carlsson, L. (2008). The Performance of Policy Networks: The Relation between Network Structure and Network Performance. *Policy Studies Journal, 36*(4), 497–524. https://doi.org/10.1111/j.1541-0072.2008.00281.x

Sandström, A., Morf, A., & Fjellborg, D. (2020). Disputed Policy Change: The Role of Events, Policy Learning, and Negotiated Agreements. *Policy Studies Journal, n/a*(n/a). doi:https://doi.org/10.1111/psj.12411

Saurugger, S. (2013). Constructivism and Public Policy Approaches in the EU: From Ideas to Power Games. *Journal of European Public Policy, 20*(6), 888–906. https://doi.org/10.1080/13501763.2013.781826

Scharpf, F. W. (1997). *Games Real Actors Play: Actor-Centered Institutionalism in Policy Research.* Westview Press.

Schlager, E. (1995). Policy Making and Collective Action: Defining Coalitions Within the Advocacy Coalition Framework. *Policy Sciences, 28*(3), 243–270. https://doi.org/10.1007/BF01000289

Schmid, N., Sewerin, S., & Schmidt, T. S. (2019). Explaining Advocacy Coalition Change with Policy Feedback. *Policy Studies Journal, 1*, 1. https://doi.org/10.1111/psj.12365

Schneider, V. (2015). Hugh Heclo, "Issue Networks and the Executive Establishment". In M. Lodge, E. C. Page, & S. J. Balla (Eds.), *The Oxford Handbook of Classics in Public Policy and Administration* (pp. 372–382). Oxford University Press.

Scott, J. (2008). Modes of Power and the Re-Conceptualization of Elites. *The Sociological Review, 56*(1_suppl), 25–43. https://doi.org/10.1111/j.1467-954X.2008.00760.x

Searing, D. D., Schwartz, J. J., & Lind, A. E. (1973). The Structuring Principle: Political Socialization and Belief Systems. *American Political Science Review,* *67*(2), 415–432. https://doi.org/10.2307/1958774

Shanahan, E. A., Jones, M. D., McBeth, M. K., & Radaelli, C. (2017). The Narrative Policy Framework. In C. M. Weible & P. A. Sabatier (Eds.), *Theories of the Policy Process* (4th ed., pp. 173–2014). Westview Press.

Shaykhutdinov, R. (2019). Socialization, Rationality, and Age: Generational Gaps and the Attitudes toward the Chechen War in Russia. *Politics & Policy, 47*(5), 931–955. https://doi.org/10.1111/polp.12323

Simon, H. A. (1947). *Administrative Behavior: A Study of Decision-Making Processes in Administrative Organization.* Free Press.

Simon, H. A. (1955). A Behavioral Model of Rational Choice. *The Quarterly Journal of Economics, 69*(1), 99–118. https://doi.org/10.2307/1884852

Simon, H. A. (1978). *Rational Decision-Making in Business Organizations.* Retrieved from

Simon, H. A. (1985). Human Nature in Politics: The Dialogue of Psychology with Political Science. *The American Political Science Review, 79*(2), 293–304.

Simon, H. A. (1990). Bounded Rationality. In J. Eatwell, M. Milgate, & P. Newman (Eds.), *Utility and Probability* (pp. 15–18). Palgrave Macmillan UK.

Simons, A., & Voß, J.-P. (2018). The Concept of Instrument Constituencies: Accounting for Dynamics and Practices of Knowing Governance. *Policy and Society, 37*(1), 14–35. https://doi.org/10.1080/14494035.2017.1375248

Skok, J. E. (1995). Policy Issue Networks and the Public Policy Cycle: A Structural-Functional Framework for Public Administration. *Public Administration Review, 55*(4), 325–332. https://doi.org/10.2307/977123

Smith, M. J. (1991). From Policy Community to Issue Network: Salmonella in Eggs and the New Politics of Food. *Public Administration, 69*(2), 235–255. https://doi.org/10.1111/j.1467-9299.1991.tb00792.x

Smith, V., & Cumming, J. (2017). Implementing Pay-for-performance in Primary Health Care: the Role of Institutional Entrepreneurs. *Policy and Society, 36*(4), 523–538. https://doi.org/10.1080/14494035.2017.1369617

Sotirov, M., & Winkel, G. (2016). Toward a Cognitive Theory of Shifting Coalitions and Policy Change: Linking the Advocacy Coalition Framework and Cultural Theory. *Policy Sciences, 49*(2), 125–154. https://doi.org/10.1007/s11077-015-9235-8

Spohr, F. (2016). Explaining Path Dependency and Deviation by Combining Multiple Streams Framework and Historical Institutionalism: A Comparative Analysis of German and Swedish Labor Market Policies. *Journal of Comparative Policy Analysis: Research and Practice, 18*(3), 257–272. https://doi.org/10.1080/13876988.2015.1122210

Steinert, C., & Yordanova, N. (2016). 'Alliance with the Enemy': Why the CDU and the Greens Formed Their First Coalition in a Large German Federal State.

German Politics, 25(1), 54–72. https://doi.org/10.1080/0964400 8.2015.1060589

Stephenson, P. J. (2010). The Role of Working Groups of Commissioners in Co-ordinating Policy Implementation: The Case of Trans-European Networks (TENs). *JCMS. Journal of Common Market Studies,* 48(3), 709–736. https://doi.org/10.1111/j.1468-5965.2010.02070.x

Stevens, A. G., Mulhollan, D. P., & Rundquist, P. S. (1981). U. S. Congressional Structure and Representation: The Role of Informal Groups. *Legislative Studies Quarterly,* 6(3), 415–437. https://doi.org/10.2307/439483

Stone, D. (2008). Global Public Policy, Transnational Policy Communities, and Their Networks. *Policy Studies Journal,* 36(1), 19–38. https://doi.org/10.1111/j.1541-0072.2007.00251.x

Strassheim, H. (2019). Behavioural Mechanisms and Public Policy Design: Preventing Failures in Behavioural Public Policy. *Public Policy and Administration,* 0952076719827062. doi:https://doi.org/10.1177/0952076719827062

Tajfel, H. (1974). Social Identity and Intergroup Behaviour. *Information (International Social Science Council),* 13(2), 65–93. https://doi.org/10.1177/053901847401300204

Tajfel, H. (1978). Social Categorization, Social Identity and Social Comparison. In H. Tajfel (Ed.), *Differentiation Between Social Groups: Studies in the Social Psychology of Intergroup Relations* (pp. 61–76). Academic Press.

Tajfel, H. (Ed.) (1982). *Social Identity and Intergroup Relations.* Cambridge Cambridgeshire; New York; Paris: Cambridge University Press; Editions de la Maison des sciences de l'homme.

Thatcher, M. (1998). The Development of Policy Network Analyses: From Modest Origins to Overarching Frameworks. *Journal of Theoretical Politics,* 10(4), 389–416. https://doi.org/10.1177/0951692898010004002

Thierse, S. (2019). Policy Entrepreneurship in the European Parliament: Reconsidering the Influence of Rapporteurs. *Journal of European Public Policy,* 26(2), 267–285. https://doi.org/10.1080/13501763.2017.1409794

Timmermans, J., van der Heiden, S., & Born, M. P. (2014). Policy Entrepreneurs in Sustainability Transitions: Their Personality and Leadership Profiles Assessed. *Environmental Innovation and Societal Transitions, 13,* 96–108. https://doi.org/10.1016/j.eist.2014.06.002

Tullia Galanti, M., & Sacchi, S. (2019). When Words Matter: Narratives and Strategies in the Italian Jobs Act (2014–2016). *Policy and Society,* 38(3), 485–501. https://doi.org/10.1080/14494035.2019.1657376

Turner, J. C. (1982). Towards a Cognitive Redefinition of a Social Group. In H. Tajfel (Ed.), *Social Identity and Intergroup Relations* (pp. 15–40). Cambridge University Press. Editions de la Maison des sciences de l'homme.

Vernardakis, G. (2013). The National School of Administration in France and Its Impact on Public Policy Making. *Croatian and Comparative Public Administration, 13*(1), 41–70.

Vogeler, C. S., Hornung, J., & Bandelow, N. C. (2020). Farm Animal Welfare Policymaking in the European Parliament – A Social Identity Perspective on Voting Behaviour. *Journal of Environmental Policy & Planning, 22*(4), 518–530.

von Beyme, K. (2001). Elite Relations in Germany. *German Politics, 10*(2), 19–36. https://doi.org/10.1080/772713261

Voß, J.-P., & Simons, A. (2014). Instrument Constituencies and the Supply Side of Policy Innovation: the Social Life of Emissions Trading. *Environmental Politics, 23*(5), 735–754. https://doi.org/10.1080/09644016.2014.923625

Wagner, P. M., & Ylä-Anttila, T. (2020). Can Policy Forums Overcome Echo Chamber Effects by Enabling Policy Learning? Evidence From the Irish climate Change Policy Network. *Journal of Public Policy, 40*(2), 194–211. https://doi.org/10.1017/S0143814X18000314

Weare, C., Lichterman, P., & Esparza, N. (2014). Collaboration and Culture: Organizational Culture and the Dynamics of Collaborative Policy Networks. *Policy Studies Journal, 42*(4), 590–619. https://doi.org/10.1111/psj.12077

Weible, C. M. (2005). Beliefs and Perceived Influence in a Natural Resource Conflict: An Advocacy Coalition Approach to Policy Networks. *Political Research Quarterly, 58*(3), 461–475. https://doi.org/10.1177/106591290505800308

Weible, C. M. (2018). Instrument Constituencies and the Advocacy Coalition Framework: An Essay on the Comparisons, Opportunities, and Intersections. *Policy and Society, 37*(1), 59–73. https://doi.org/10.1080/1449403 5.2018.1417705

Weible, C. M., Ingold, K., Nohrstedt, D., Henry, A. D., & Jenkins-Smith, H. C. (2019). Sharpening Advocacy Coalitions. *Policy Studies Journal, 1*, 2. https://doi.org/10.1111/psj.12360

Weible, C. M., & Nohrstedt, D. (2012). The Advocacy Coalition Framework: Coalitions, Learning and Policy Change. In E. Araral, S. Fritzen, M. Howlett, M. Ramesh, & X. Wu (Eds.), *Routledge Handbook of Public Policy* (pp. 125–137). Routledge.

Weible, C. M., Sabatier, P. A., & McQueen, K. (2009). Themes and Variations: Taking Stock of the Advocacy Coalition Framework. *Policy Studies Journal, 37*(1), 121–140. https://doi.org/10.1111/j.1541-0072.2008.00299.x

Weiner, S., & Tatum, D. S. (2020). Rethinking Identity in Political Science. *Political Studies Review, 1478929920919360*. https://doi.org/10.1177/1478929920919360

Weinschenk, A. C. (2017). Big Five Personality Traits, Political Participation, and Civic Engagement: Evidence from 24 Countries. *Social Science Quarterly, 98*(5), 1406–1421. https://doi.org/10.1111/ssqu.12380

Wellstead, A. (2017). Plus ça Change, Plus C'est La Même Chose? A Review of Paul Sabatier's "An Advocacy Coalition Framework of Policy Change and the Role of Policy-Oriented Learning Therein". *Policy Sciences, 50*(4), 549–561. https://doi.org/10.1007/s11077-017-9307-z

Wenzelburger, G. (2015). Parties, Institutions and the Politics of Law and Order: How Political Institutions and Partisan Ideologies Shape Law-and-Order Spending in Twenty Western Industrialized Countries. *British Journal of Political Science, 45*(3), 663–687. https://doi.org/10.1017/S0007123413000501

Wildavsky, A. (1964). *The Politics of the Budgetary Process.* Little, Brown.

Wilson, C. A. (2000). Policy Regimes and Policy Change. *Journal of Public Policy, 20*(3), 247–274. https://doi.org/10.1017/S0143814X00000842

Witting, A., & Dudley, G. (2020). A Long-term Perspective on Entrepreneurial Strategies and Their Impact on British Road Policy. *European Policy Analysis, 6*(1), 58–76. https://doi.org/10.1002/epa2.1070

Wu, C.-I., & Lin, A. M.-W. (2019). Do Cohorts Matter? Cohort Analysis and Value-Difference Impressions of a Rising China. *Political Studies Review, 17*(4), 391–415. https://doi.org/10.1177/1478929919864781

Yagci, A. H. (2019). Policy Knowledge, Collective Action and Advocacy Coalitions: Regulating GMOs in Turkey. *Journal of European Public Policy, 26*(6), 927–945. https://doi.org/10.1080/13501763.2018.1509884

Zafonte, M., & Sabatier, P. A. (1998). Shared Beliefs and Imposed Interdependencies as Determinants of Ally Networks in Overlapping Subsystems. *Journal of Theoretical Politics, 10*(4), 473–505. https://doi.org/10.1177/0951692898010004005

Zahariadis, N. (2003). *Ambiguity and Choice in Public Policy: Political Decision Making in Modern Democracies.* Georgetown University Press.

Zahariadis, N. (2016). Bounded Rationality and Garbage Can Models of Policy-Making. In B. G. Peters & P. Zittoun (Eds.), *Contemporary Approaches to Public Policy: Theories, Controversies and Perspectives* (pp. 155–174). Palgrave Macmillan UK.

Zahariadis, N., & Exadaktylos, T. (2016). Policies that Succeed and Programs that Fail: Ambiguity, Conflict, and Crisis in Greek Higher Education. *Policy Studies Journal, 44*(1), 59–82. https://doi.org/10.1111/psj.12129

Zito, A. R. (2018). Instrument Constituencies and Epistemic Community Theory. *Policy and Society, 37*(1), 36–58. https://doi.org/10.1080/14494035.2017.1416929

Zohlnhöfer, R. (2016). Putting Together the Pieces of the Puzzle: Explaining German Labor Market Reforms with a Modified Multiple-Streams Approach. *Policy Studies Journal, 44*(1), 83–107. https://doi.org/10.1111/psj.12135

Zohlnhöfer, R., Herweg, N., & Huß, C. (2016). Bringing Formal Political Institutions into the Multiple Streams Framework: An Analytical Proposal for Comparative Policy Analysis. *Journal of Comparative Policy Analysis: Research and Practice*, *18*(3), 243–256. https://doi.org/10.1080/1387698 8.2015.1095428

Zohlnhöfer, R., & Rüb, F. W. (Eds.). (2016). *Decision-Making Under Ambiguity and Time Constraints: Assessing the Multiple-Streams Framework*. ECPR Press.

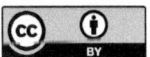

CHAPTER 3

Political Institutions and Public Policy

In order to shed light on this missing link between programmatic action and political institutions, this chapter reviews how institutions are currently discussed in policy process research in order to derive hypotheses that may explain under which institutional conditions programmatic action should or should not take place. The goal of this overview of the state of the art is twofold. On the one hand, it serves to assess the contribution of the PAF to existing theories of the policy process and the understanding of institutions in it. In doing so, it becomes clear why a new theoretical lens is needed and where and why the PAF is able to fill gaps left by others. On the other hand, the established approaches to explaining policy change and stability with respect to policy processes contain assumptions and hypotheses about the role of institutions that can be integrated into the PAF and help sharpen the analytical power of a look at the institutional conditions for programmatic action. They do this by formulating mechanisms between theoretical concepts that can also be adapted, or at least assumed to be relevant, to the formation of programmatic groups and the success of the group and its program. At the very least, they lay the groundwork for the question that asks about the influence of institutional settings familiar in comparative politics on policy change.

With these two goals in mind, the following chapters systematically review the state of the art based on five main lines of literature and with a

© The Author(s) 2022
J. Hornung, *The Institutions of Programmatic Action,*
International Series on Public Policy,
https://doi.org/10.1007/978-3-031-05774-8_3

particular focus on institutions. Overviews of theories of the policy process have been published in the form of textbooks in various languages (Maillard & Kübler, 2015; Schubert & Bandelow, 2014; Weible & Sabatier, 2017; Wenzelburger & Zohlnhöfer, 2015) and serve as an initial source to identify the sample considered here. What is innovative about the PAF and previously neglected in these textbooks is the focus on long-term periods of programmatic stability in policy change, traced back to programmatic groups and the social psychological explanation of individual behavior as the basis for collective action and resulting policy change. When one thinks of explanations for programmatic stability, institutionalist theories immediately come to mind. Thus, a first look at the research focuses on explanations for policy stability. This begins with institutional explanations of federalism and veto players and continues by examining the involvement of different interests in the policy-making process, for example, through corporatist structures or public protest. A particular emphasis is then placed on the role of bureaucratic recruitment and policy advice, as these institutions are assumed to be particularly relevant to programmatic action.

However, before beginning with the outlined theoretical groundwork, it is necessary to define institutions as they are to be understood from a PAF perspective. In political science, a general distinction is made between a broader and a narrower understanding of institutions, with the narrower understanding commonly associated with the "old institutionalism" (Peters, 1996). Within the neo-institutionalist tradition, institutions are defined by looking at the influence they exert on actors and thus include the informal rules that guide actors' behavior (Wenzelburger & Zohlnhöfer, 2014, p. 314). The PAF uses a broader understanding of institutions as not only the rules governing behavior, but also the existence of agencies and organizations that shape the interaction between individuals and thus contribute to group formation and group action. This view likewise includes institutions that can stand in the way of programmatic groups as they seek to translate their program into policy decisions. In this way, the definition is similar to that of March and Olsen (2008, pp. 4-5) that institutions are determined by repetitive processes that need to be explored in terms of their effect on individuals and the resulting institutional stability (Capano, 2018), and that institutions (rules, but also agencies and social systems) are also carriers of identities that influence policy actors.

3.1 Veto Players and Federalism

Institutionalist analysis is closely related to the notion of which institutions impede or enable change. In comparative politics, institutional analysis is often linked to whether the political system is parliamentary or presidential, although the usefulness of this dichotomy for analyzing institutions is debatable (Cheibub et al., 2014). Essentially, the difference is whether or not the government is dependent on parliament, such that parliament can remove the government. It has been argued previously that the apparent balance between cabinet and parliament is symbolic rather than politically relevant because of the interdependence of offices and support on both sides (Price, 1943, p. 319). From an office-seeking perspective, the parliament will do everything possible to avoid dissolution and new elections. In presidential systems such as the US, the cabinet and parliament are separate and independent because of independent elections. The archetype of semi-presidentialism was developed by Maurice Duverger with reference to France, although it is controversial whether France can be considered this semi-presidential archetype (Elgie, 2009) and French political scientists reject this typology (Pasquino, 2005).

Among the various typologies in comparative politics is that of Arend Lijphart (2012), who differentiates patterns of democracy based on two dimensions. These dimensions consider, first, executive capacity, including party systems, cabinet functioning, legislative-executive relations, electoral systems, interest groups, and, on a second dimension, the degree of federal or unitary organization of politics. The extent to which these institutions contribute to or prevent policy change is a matter of debate. Pierson (1995, p. 472) outlines the various interaction effects that federalist structures have on social policy change.

In part because of this complexity, which makes it difficult to compare analyses across different political systems, veto player theory has emerged as an alternative lens on institutions (Tsebelis, 2002). Rather than analyzing the entire institutional setting of a given political system and its consequences for policy making, this approach is interested only in those institutional actors that are necessary to change the status quo (Tsebelis, 2000, p. 442). Institutional veto players are metonymic with veto points (Immergut, 2006, p. 568). They describe the very institutions that are mandatorily involved in adopting a policy. When within an institutional veto player, multiple parties are required for a majority decision, they are referred to as partisan veto players (Tsebelis, 1995, p. 302f). Since the work of George Tsebelis, there has been an increasing number of studies on veto players and their power that test the five main hypotheses of veto player theory (C. Jensen & Wenzelburger, 2020; Wenzelburger, 2011; Zohlnhöfer, 2003). These postulate that the greater the number of veto players, the more cohesive they are, the greater the ideological distance between the veto players and between the current and previous governments, and the shorter the duration of government, the less likely a change in the status quo will occur (Schmidt, 2002, p. 152). In this regard, research provides evidence on the relationship between veto players government types (Angelova et al., 2018), institution-building (Hallerberg, 2011), globalization pressures (Ha, 2007), international trade policy and the change in tariffs (O'Reilly, 2005), the rule of law (Andrews & Montinola, 2004), budget composition (Tsebelis & Chang, 2004), and many others. In recent years, research also indicates that legal actors are conditional veto players depending on whether their preferences are absorbed by another institutional veto player (Brouard & Hönnige, 2017). In order to assess the institutional settings in the two most different contexts in this respect—France and Germany—the institutional and partisan veto players in these states are reviewed below.

For parliamentary systems, among which he also classes France, Tsebelis (1999, p. 593f) argues that, in addition to the governing parties, the second body of the legislative arena or the head of state could potentially be considered veto players. Since the French president, as head of state, has some veto power over government decrees, he could be seen as an institutional veto player only in times of divided government. However, Tsebelis (1995, p. 306) also emphasizes France as an exceptional case in which a strong president and a bicameral legislative system are de facto coded as a system with only one institutional veto player, namely the National Assembly (NA). Since the beginning of the Fifth Republic in 1958, French parliamentarism has been described as rationalized for several reasons. One is the government's ability to have bills voted on as a package vote; a second is its ability to combine a vote on a bill with a vote of confidence (Hayward, 2004, p. 83). Other limitations include the government's ability to rule by decree, to set the parliamentary agenda, and the degradation of the parliamentary committees (Keeler, 1993, p. 521f). Another is the lack of a comprehensive right to introduce amendments to bills. Navarro, Vaillant, and Wolff (2012, pp. 58/74) argue that the constitutional reform in 2008 gave greater weight to committee work, in which those who hold multiple offices, in particular, attend meetings regularly, contribute efficiently to tabling legislative amendments, and provide oversight of the government. The reform also strengthened the role of parliament by limiting the president's ability to couple proposals with a vote of confidence and to require parliamentary approval for certain foreign and domestic policy decisions (Michel, 2008). Now, amendments to bills most often come from the government or parliamentary committees and are also more successful when introduced in committees than in parliament (Kerrouche, 2006, pp. 355-357). It can be concluded that the legislative arena of the National Assembly in France is of particular importance with regard to parliamentary committees, which have a special relationship to the respective ministers (Fasone, 2017, p. 16).

Given that the constitutional amendment in 2008 also allowed the opposition to initiate an abstract review, the Conseil Constitutionnel (constitutional council) was strengthened as a potentially second institutional veto player. Unlike comparable institutions in other countries, the Conseil Constitutionnel is able to exert influence during the legislative process and is therefore quite powerful; it can decide that legislative texts are not in conformity with the constitution and, on this basis, delete parts of legislative texts (François, 1997). With the 2008 reform, it is now also able to retroactively declare laws unconstitutional. In general, however, Brouard (2009) describes constitutional vetoes as electorally incentivized and politicized. They have been used primarily in electoral competition to signal positions to voters and to control the government (Brouard, 2009, p. 386/396). The Conseil Constitutionnel thus represents a conditional veto player, depending on its ideological composition (Brouard & Hönnige, 2017).

A key feature of French semi-presidentialism is the divided executive, where the prime minister sits in parliament and the president resides in the Elysée Palace without having the right to enter the NA. As a rule, the relationship between the president and the prime minister, whom he appoints as well as the ministers of the cabinet (after nomination by the previously appointed prime minister), is cooperative. Since there are only a few months between NA elections and presidential elections, the winning political party is in most cases the same—but only since the 2002 institutional reform (Grossman & Sauger, 2009). Scholars have argued that there is an institutional presidential bias in the sense that the ability to reshuffle governments gives the president dominance over the prime minister in intra-party relations and an opportunity for blame avoidance, but this does not seem to work well (Grossman, 2009, p. 277). Presidential dominance does not stop with the government, but usually extends to the majority party in parliament (Cole, 1993, p. 63). However, dominance over the majority in parliament can tip, especially when the parties securing the majority are in conflict (Lazardeux, 2009, p. 288) and when ideological distance within parliamentary coalitions is significant, weakening party unity in voting (Godbout & Foucault, 2013, p. 324). Indeed, while the prime minister and cabinet are in a weaker institutional position because they need the backing of parliament and the president, the centralization of power at the presidential level makes the president the main figure of accountability and provides fewer opportunities for coalition building to share blame (Bezes & Le Lidec, 2015, p. 502). In the face of strong opposition in parliament, both enacted and failed legislation lower the executive's popularity (Becher & Brouard, 2020). Finally, regarding this institutional setting in France, the government's relationship with the president, as well as with parliament, should not be underestimated when explaining reform success.

If the president and prime minister do not share party affiliation, this constitutes divided government, known as cohabitation. Here, the prime minister's power again depends on the majority in parliament and is linked to whether the majority party expects electoral success in the upcoming elections, which would place the prime minister as a likely presidential candidate (Lazardeux, 2015, p. 88). In terms of legislative efficiency, which is supposed to be lower under divided governments because of the risk of gridlock, productivity levels actually do not differ significantly between divided and unified governments because actors are able to cooperate, but major structural reforms are more likely under a unified government (Baumgartner et al., 2014, p. 444).

Another type of divided government exists in the case of different majorities in the Senate and the NA. Nevertheless, the Senate is not considered a true veto player, since in case of disagreement on a bill, a mediation committee is convened. After its report, however, the NA still has the final decision-making power, so the Senate can delay a law but not prevent it. However, since the Senate in France is indirectly elected, it is mainly local representatives who sit in the Senate, which often reflects the conflict between the national government and local governments, especially the Assembly of Mayors (Assemblée des Maires de France).

German federalism entails the institution of the Federal Council (Bundesrat), which is involved in the legislative process. Although not all laws are subject to the explicit approval of the Bundesrat, it is an institutional veto player for those that are, and especially in policy areas that affect Länder interests (Zohlnhöfer, 2003, p. 130). In health policy, this concerns, among others things, hospital policy (since it is within the competence of the Länder to bear the investment costs for hospitals), emergency care, and regionally active sickness funds (Dent et al., 2004, p. 732). Thus, the Bundesrat represents a second institutional veto player in addition to the governing parties. Moreover, it can be argued that the degree of cohesion within the veto players is higher, at least as far as the parties are concerned. This is not because there are no intra-party conflicts in Germany, as a number of studies confirm (Debus & Bräuninger, 2008; Marx & Schumacher, 2013; Seeleib-Kaiser, 2010; Steiner & Mader, 2017), but because legislative processes in Germany are dominated by the parliamentary parties of the governing coalition, and MPs are rarely freed from the obligation to vote in accordance with parliamentary party policy. Even then, party membership exerts a significant influence on individual preferences (Engler & Dümig, 2017). Since the Bundesrat consists of representatives of the Länder governments, and a Land's vote can only be cast unanimously, the Bundesrat is sometimes misused for party-political and intra-coalitional conflict (Auel, 2014, p. 425; Brunner & Debus, 2008; Lehmbruch, 1998).

The term divided government is also used to describe divergent party-political majorities in the Bundestag and Bundesrat, which is also said to have a negative impact on legislative productivity (Manow & Burkhart, 2011). Similar to France, a constitutional reform was designed to increase the power of parliament, but in the German case at the expense of the power of the Bundesrat (Stecker, 2016). In historical retrospect, though, Germany is characterized as a grand coalition state that permits governing only in coalitions between parties as well as between the federal and the state level (Schmidt, 2008, p. 90). Empirical testing of these contradictory views found evidence of dynamic patterns of policy-making and mixed results for both competitive and consensual policy-making with respect to the policy domain (Breunig, 2014, p. 144). When party coalition dominance differs in the Bundestag and Bundesrat, votes in the Bundesrat are sometimes won by concessions regarding state interests (Ganghof & Bräuninger, 2006, p. 533). Thus, divided government also contributes to a more consensus-oriented relationship between government and opposition in the Bundestag at the outset of legislative initiatives (Hohendorf et al., 2020). Summarizing the relationship between the Bundestag and the Bundesrat, then, one can conclude that both represent arenas that are heavily dominated by party groups and regional interests. The subnational level of government should not be neglected in the policy-making process.

The German government consists of the chancellor and his/her cabinet members, who are politicians appointed by the chancellor, who in turn sets guidelines and organizes the executive branch (Müller-Rommel, 1997, p. 172). Coalition governments at the federal level have always consisted of up to three parties, although the increasing success of the right-wing Alternative for Germany (Alternative für Deutschland, AfD) is challenging the existing party system and making two-party coalitions less likely (Bräuninger et al., 2019, p. 83). A central and, in recent years, increasing role in legislation at the local, regional, and national levels is attributed to the coalition agreement on which the government-forming parties agree (Gross & Krauss, 2019). In this context, the content of such coalition agreements often includes conflict issues on which the parties try to make as few concessions as possible to their respective coalition partners (Klüver & Bäck, 2019). However, this is not always the case, and even the most ideologically distant coalitions can govern cooperatively if the portfolio allocation and sites of conflict resolution are strategically chosen (Saalfeld et al., 2019). The head of state has no veto power and only a representative function, but becomes important in crisis situations such as a lack of parliamentary majority for chancellor and government formation (Hornung et al., 2020).

The systematic analysis of veto players in the two countries helps identify key positions that programmatic groups need to cover—or will aim to cover—to ensure minimal resistance to the implementation of their policy program. This mechanism is similar to that proposed by the veto control hypothesis in analyses of cabinet formation (Eppner & Ganghof, 2017). Thus, the PAF actually draws on and incorporates institutional factors that help or hinder the formation and success of "new alliances" (Hacker, 2004, p. 718). Horizontal collaboration at the local level may prove to be a necessary element in paving the way for major policy change and path dependencies (Hager & Hamagami, 2020). Given the above considerations, the importance of the subnational level of policy-making depends on the degree of federalism. As a consequence, it can be expected that:

Decentralization Hypothesis
In decentralized democracies, the involvement of subnational actors is a necessary condition for programmatic group formation. The involvement of subnational actors then also is necessary for programmatic groups' success.

In addition to veto players, which can potentially prevent and block reforms, health policy decision-making processes in France and Germany are also shaped by other institutions that can directly influence decision-making. Unlike in the case of veto players, however, this influence is not mandatory. The following chapter therefore focuses on corporatist structures as distinct loci of decision-making, which are also most relevant to health policy.

3.2   Corporatism and Organized Interests

Mediation between collective interests and the state is usually subsumed under the research strands of pluralism, lobbyism, and corporatism (Klenk, 2018, p. 21). Schmitter (1974), in his widely cited state of the art article, defines corporatism as

> *a system of interest and/or attitude representation, a particular modal or ideal-typical institutional arrangement for linking the associationally organized interests of civil society with the decisional structures of the state. (Schmitter, 1974, p. 86)*

In the course of further research, scholars have drawn a distinction between a structural understanding of corporatism (as defined above) and a processual understanding that places more emphasis on the process of policy-making from agenda setting and formulation to implementation. The latter is labeled concertation, while the combination of the two is called neo-corporatism (Baccaro, 2003, p. 685). Similarly, Lehmbruch (1977, p. 95) emphasizes that interests are not only linked and integrated into the policy process, but that interest associations are in effect given responsibility for specific decisions and their implementation, which emphasizes the reciprocal dimension of linkage. Critics argue that the de facto primacy of the state interest over sectoral interests persists and that this even diminishes the earlier competition between interest groups to lobby in the policy process (Cox, 1981, p. 79). Nonetheless, the degree to which interests are involved in the policy process in terms of ensuring compliance with the enacted reforms and providing tying knots for organized groups is an important feature for this study's interest in explaining collective action in the policy process and programmatic change.

Corporatism has been shown to be a component of consensus democracy (Lijphart & Crepaz, 1991, p. 245) and, although this view has been challenged (Keman & Pennings, 1995, p. 279), has been incorporated in the comparative politics typology of democracies by Lijphart (2012). France and Germany differ most in terms of the relationship between the state and interest groups, both regarding regular exchange and systematic involvement in the processes of policy formulation and adoption. In Germany, recurrent forms of exchange between the state and interest groups in the form of consultations represent a new type of negotiation democracy (Czada, 2015). In France, on the other hand, corporatist arrangements, which are institutionalized forms of governance, are not realized even though there is a willingness on the part of the respective unions and associations to do so and even though there is a need to address financial pressures, including through pro-capital policies and the intro-duction of competitive elements (Lux, 2015). This is not to say that unions in France do not have some influence on the parliamentary process and that their strikes would not have a significant impact (Mazevet et al., 2018; Weßels, 2007, p. 110).

Many studies in corporatism have focused on the economic and labor market sectors (Heinze & Schmid, 1997; Parsons, 1988). When corporat-ism refers only to a sectoral alignment of interests and agreement, the term meso-corporatism is usually used (Cawson, 1985). Molina and Rhodes (2002, p. 326) argue for a process-oriented rather than a structure-oriented understanding of corporatism, focusing on actor networks rather than formal institutions. An important aspect for the development of actor networks from corporatist structures is the exclusivity with which associa-tions have a monopoly position in negotiating agreements with the state (Klenk, 2018, p. 22).

With respect to the health sector, corporatist elements are strongly exis-tent in Germany and also present—but to a different degree—in France. The French and German health care reforms in the 1990s had a structural and in some cases negative impact on the actors of self-governance and medical professions. In particular, the inherent goal of cost containment is not attractive to corporatist actors (Godt, 1987). However, the physicians' associations in both countries were unable to prevent these reforms (Hassenteufel, 1997, pp. 8-9). Following on from the executive-legislative relations outlined earlier, the declining influence of these interest groups in France can be explained by the parliamentary backing of the govern-ment in the absence of cohabitation in 1995, the lack of which had previ-ously provided opportunities for interest group influence (Immergut, 1990, p. 397). The strongest organized interest group in the French health care system is physicians, who value their elitist status, resulting from many years of top-level training and a numerus clausus (not abolished until 2019), and protect it against state interventions (Mendy, 2015, p. 9). Some scholars even argue that the group of physicians has political and economic resources that outweigh any formal institutional rules and grant bargaining power in any state (Marmor & Thomas, 1972, p. 438). While the lack of involvement of corporatist actors in the policy process in France allows for a more centralized state-led policy process, primarily through administrative, statist regulation, which has been positively associated with the effectiveness of cost containment measures (Wilsford, 1991), this also presents a downside for health policy-making in France. The high political costs and the manifest opposition, which, although it has fewer means of institutionalized decision-making power, represents a stiff resistance to reforms can only be addressed by centralized hierarchical administrative governance (Hassenteufel, 1996, p. 478). Medical entrepreneurs who aim to shape policy, however, become a grateful type of ally for state actors to drive new reforms (Hassenteufel et al., 2020, p. 54). Thus, it is not straightforward to derive a strength or weakness of the state from corporatist structures, as both views have their justification (von Beyme, 1983, p. 177).

In contrast, Germany has a tradition of corporatist structures and self-governing bodies in the health care system, which means that the welfare associations are assigned tasks and, in some cases, regulatory powers in a reciprocal working relationship with the state (Toens, 2008, p. 102). A key feature of the German health care system is the indirect role of elected officials in the financing and provision of health care services, the responsibility for which is shifted to the self-governance of health care actors (Saltman, 1997, p. S17). The success of a far-reaching health policy reform in Germany in 1992, after almost 50 years of blocking of major reforms by interest groups, can be attributed to a grand coalition compromise (Bandelow, 1998, p. 210). In parallel with the reforms in France, cost containment measures were enforced that had previously been in force but with which the associations of statutory health insurance physicians (Kassenärztliche Vereinigungen, KV) had not previously complied (Giaimo, 1995, p. 364f). Since then, the influence of interest groups has depended heavily on the substantive and discursive congruence of their interests with the politically dominant guiding principles (Bandelow, 2007a, p. 290). On the other hand, the reform also maintained and intentionally strengthened collective agreements negotiated between the social partners (Giaimo & Manow, 1999, p. 978). This can be seen as a first sign of the centralization of competences that progressed in the 2000s and led to a selective strengthening of the competences of certain bodies of self-governance and joint decision-making, while holistically it tended to erode established corporatist structures (Gerlinger, 2010, p. 127f). Recent analyses assess these changes as a dismantling of the established German welfare state model (Trampusch, 2020, p. 159f).

To summarize the institutional perspective of corporatism in terms of its influence on the core interest of this book, programmatic groups and policy programs, there are two concluding observations that will be considered in the following. First, it can be questioned whether corporatist arrangements generally lead to more or less legislative productivity or state effectiveness. Delegating central government decision-making authority to the interest association level offers the advantage of a more cooperative style of policy-making with less substantive and public resistance to reform, but at the same time requires the need for compromise. Following this observation, recent research recommends taking into account the specific institutional environment to assess its relevance (Giuliani, 2016, p. 38). From the perspective of the veto player control hypothesis, regardless of the exact degree of corporatism in a given country, it may be helpful to coordinate legislative proposals with interest associations to gain support and keep opposition low. To this end, and similar to what Bandelow calls discursive alignment (Bandelow, 2007a, p. 290), it is useful to choose a narrative or discursive frame for policy reforms that fits the interests of the relevant stakeholders. In line with the previous considerations on veto players, high delegation of power to self-governing bodies in the health care system could therefore be seen as creating sectoral veto players that can collectively block policies through delayed or misguided implementation. Corporatism also provides a complementary perspective to explain opportunities for group formation and to reveal actors potentially forming joint reform alliances, as meso-corporatism usually provides institutionalized opportunities for exchange (von Winter, 2014, p. 179). One would therefore expect that:

Self-Governance Hypothesis
When competencies are delegated to self-governance of sectoral actors, it is necessary for programmatic action to occur that programmatic actors either emerge from self-governance or that programmatic groups encompass actors from the self-governance to be successful.

Sectoral actors do this either by putting forward policy proposals themselves, forming alliances with or without state actors, or publicly opposing reforms and using narratives to generate acceptance for their views. The ways in which a political system introduces interests either through sectoral actors or the public thereby helps to examine the extent to which such structures influence the process of group formation and what types of groups emerge.

While citizens rarely have direct means of influence, the culture of protest in France is exceptionally strong, as demonstrated most recently by the protests of the so-called yellow vests (Chamorel, 2019). In addition to elections in which they vote for the president and the NA, citizens participate in political debates often through public demonstrations in major cities. One example of extra-parliamentary participation is the "Grand Débat" (great debate) initiated by then-president Emmanuel Macron in early 2019 in response to yellow vests protests against the government. While the government set the overarching themes of ecological transition, taxes/expenditure, state organization, and democracy/citizenship, health policy emerged as another issue on citizens' side, especially regarding access to health care (Tranthimy, 2019). Thus, while French policy-makers do not face strong blockage of reforms by powerful corporate actors, they do face the challenge of legitimizing reforms to the French public, which, not least because of the party system, indicates a crisis of representation (Shields, 2005). This is not limited to France, as research on the impact of protests on legislative agendas in Western countries, including Germany, shows that protests have an impact, especially on social welfare issues. However, this effect is said to be stronger in majoritarian than in consensus democracies (Bernardi et al., 2020, p. 16f).

3.3 BUREAUCRATIC RECRUITMENT SYSTEMS AND ELITE BUILDING

Elite studies have a long tradition of examining what makes individuals elites and what influence elites have on society and political decisions. Probably the most prominent works are by Mills (2000) and Robert Dahl (1961), whose work is also referred to by Genieys and Hassenteufel (2012). The principle derived from this work, that elites can be identified through a "decisional approach" because they are found in formal decision-making positions, is also the basis of the PAF. There is a general consensus on the definition of elites as political actors with a substantial influence on decision-making (Hoffmann-Lange, 2007, p. 910). But how do actors reach these positions? To assess the likelihood of programmatic group formation in different countries, it is essential to review the education systems of elite recruiting. Knowing which career paths lead to power (i.e., positions in the policy-making process) enables researchers to know where programmatic groups will form and which channels to monitor and merge to trigger programmatic action. The empirical study informed the answer to this question through systematic biographical analyses of programmatic actors. It has been shown that the elite system in France differs from that in Germany.

The elite system in France is essentially shaped by the institution of the ENA and its associated career paths. Actuaries trained in this institution are not only placed in the top positions of administration and politics, they also already form informal networks among themselves, which have a long-term impact on their work (Searls, 1978, p. 171). Thus, the structures in France are much more elite than in Germany; Suleiman Suleiman (1974) also refers to these key actors as the administrative elite. In health policy, Genieys and Smyrl (2008, p. 80) find these actors in the Grand Corps and IGAS, as well as in the central administration of sickness funds. While the path to these positions in France almost exclusively through the ENA, career paths in Germany are more diverse.

Since as early as the eighteenth century, the recruitment processes of senior civil servants in Germany have proceeded through university routes, originally with a strong focus on law studies, which later opened up to social sciences and economics as alternative entry levels into the senior civil service (Derlien, 1991, p. 392). In the case of German health policy, empirical analysis has linked the emergence of programmatic action to the rise of health economists in the system, which contributed essentially to the establishment of a network among these actors (Ulrich, 2012). At the same time, even below the level of politicians, partisanship is a relevant determinant of careers not only in the policy-making process (Bach & Veit, 2018; Kube, 2004). Research from other parliamentary countries such as Portugal shows that career paths that run through parties are more durable than those that run only through the civil service or parliament (Seixas & Costa, 2021). Parties should therefore not be neglected when it comes to the formation of elites. Although electoral programs and party manifestos are distinct from the concept of policy programs as defined by the PAF, one hypothesis could also be that parties in parliamentary systems take on the task of program generation, which rather makes nations with less stable party systems form programmatic groups as an alternative venue for idea generation.

In terms of integrating political elite studies into public policy research, there has been little but important research on how the recruitment of elites and their role in policy processes differs across countries, but how accounting for these differences can inform political science (Blondel & Müller-Rommel, 2007). This is not to say that elite studies in general have a young history; the work of Mills and Dahl and the seminal work of Putnam (1976) prove otherwise. They already saw a small group of elite individuals, characterized by professional and biographical backgrounds and sectoral specialization, as predisposing to influence in a policy area. Yet public policy research and policy processes have placed less emphasis on a systematic examination of individual elite actors and how the structures of elite recruitment as institutional predispositions shape pathways to policy change. This is where the PAF comes in and fills a gap by focusing on elite formation and the construction of elite groups. *The 2018 Palgrave Handbook of Political Elites*, which summarizes the current state of elite research worldwide (Best & Higley, 2018), provides fruitful insights in this regard. Summarizing research on "executive elites", Verzichelli (2018) notes that each state is typically led by a small group of executive-elite actors who share a kind of history that binds them together and is characterized by specific relationships between those who come from the political field and those who come from the administrative field of work. The political-administrative relationship is not only a crucial aspect in defining elites, but also in their collaboration, as will become clearer in the following subchapter on the science-policy nexus.

Building on these findings of elite research in public policy, the question arises as to what makes individuals members of elite groups and how they can become programmatic actors. In this regard, the PAF provides a possible link between the often separately discussed background and behavior of elite actors (Rhodes et al., 2007, p. 5). Highlighting the role of the education systems and career paths institutionalized in the ENA as elite-forming institutions in France and the field of study and respective political and sectoral career paths as elite-forming institutions in Germany, the following hypothesis is formulated:

Biographical Identity Hypothesis
Programmatic action depends on the existence of institutions that foster shared biographies among actors and thus favor group formation.

Generalizing these institutional conditions, one can conclude that there are functional analogies in the institutions that produce top policy actors and that identifying them is an important step in finding potential programmatic actors. However, research also confirms that not only the professional background but also membership in relevant legislative bodies are predisposing factors for the generation of innovative ideas (Makse, 2020). The hypothesis includes the understanding that the institution relevant for programmatic action is the presence of elite formation structures that establish commonalities among actors, be it the same education, the same partisan ideology, or the same work environment (ministry, sickness fund, or other state-related institution). Structures of elite formation favor the formation of groups because they ensure a common background among policy actors.

3.4   Policy Advice and Scientific Impulses

If it can be assumed that social groups are formed on the basis of shared characteristics and that these groups influence the policy process over time, the question arises as to what drives their innovative ideas and the promotions during the policy process. In terms of PAF, ideas are compiled into what is called a policy program, and this program is said to reflect in part the policy preferences of the programmatic actors, but it cannot be seen as a mere translation of preexisting preferences or even beliefs into policy. But where do these ideas come from? In general, they can be either externally borrowed, that is, transferred from other political systems and following other national and international experiences (exogenous generation of policy ideas), or generated from within a policy subsystem, for example, by expert commissions, evaluations, or scientific results produced by think tanks and national universities (endogenous generation of scientific knowledge).

A focus on the exogenous generation of policy ideas profits from the review of literature on policy transfer and internationalization in explaining the adoption of certain reform strategies from other governments. This literature clearly distinguishes between policy innovation and policy invention, with the latter describing the original development of new policy instruments and the former referring to the adoption of policy instruments from other jurisdictions or systems (Berry & Berry, 2017, p. 253f). There are four most prominent mechanisms of policy diffusion (Shipan & Volden, 2008) organized around the three main dynamics of voluntary adoption of policies from other countries, regulatory race, and external pressure and coercion to adopt policies. The first dimension here subsumes two mechanisms that were originally separate in the literature, imitation, and learning, as these are difficult to disentangle empirically.

The first part of the policy transfer and diffusion models sheds light on the processes by which governments learn from the experiences of other countries by idealizing them as role models, imitating them, or deliberately following different paths. When transferring policies—where it is often not clear whether they imitate other countries to create an ingroup feeling or whether they have actually learned from the experiences of foreign governments—an important assessment relates to the integration of policies developed for and in different institutional contexts into the respective institutional setting (referred to as institutional fit) (Obinger et al., 2013, p. 122f). Whether policies fit institutional settings depends on policy-related and institutional characteristics. Thus, from which countries governments adopt policies depends on a number of factors (Maggetti & Gilardi, 2016, p. 93). Similar institutional settings can favor policy adoption (Strang & Meyer, 1993), as can the preexistence of certain cultural values (J. L. Jensen, 2003). Similarly, geographically and ideologically close ("neighboring") systems are more likely to learn from each other (Grossback et al., 2004; Mertens et al., 2019, p. 14; Mitchell, 2018). The ideological argument also applies to the imitation of political parties by their transnational counterparts (Wolkenstein et al., 2019) and a party-based propensity to adopt ideologically different policies (Butler et al., 2017). A prominent example is the third way politics in labor parties worldwide, most notably promoted by Tony Blair (Johnson & Tonkiss, 2002).

Secondly, the competitive nature of policy transfer and diffusion is inherently trying to perform not just as good as other countries (as suggested by learning or imitation argument), but better than others, especially in relation to the global market (Marsh & Sharman, 2009, pp. 271-272). In doing so, governments may seek to make themselves more attractive in terms of tax policy (Burge & Rogers, 2016) and align their policies accordingly in the competition for businesses' locations (Baybeck et al., 2011; Leiser, 2015). Whether these processes lead to higher or lower standards in comparative regulation is summarized under terms such as races to the top and races to the bottom. Following this debate, scholars have noted a race to the top in, for example, environmental standards (Bastiaens & Postnikov, 2017; Busch et al., 2005, p. 164; Saikawa, 2013) and a race to the bottom in higher education spending (Bailey et al., 2004, p. 72), as well as mixed results in labor rights (Mosley & Uno, 2007).

Thirdly, increasing processes of internationalization have led states to adopt policies because they would otherwise fear sanctions. Such coercive policy diffusion is only possible if international organizations or supranational institutions (such as the EU) have the necessary threat potential to force states to adopt policies. Alternatively, states can credibly exchange support or cooperation for policy adoption and attach policy adoption as a condition of action. Processes of policy adoption through coercion or pressure can be distinguished from harmonized intentions to converge policies and from more uncoordinated mechanisms of policy diffusion (Busch & Jörgens, 2005, p. 867). Among relatively equivalent states in terms of economic performance, demographics, and import/export relations, coercion is more likely to be exerted in the course of treaty formation (Morin & Gold, 2014, p. 784). Alternatively, there is political pressure under which public sector organizations reform to maintain the flow of support and resources (Andersen & Jakobsen, 2018, p. 217). A prominent example is the case of Greece, which was forced to implement austerity measures in exchange for financial aid during the financial and economic crisis (Obinger et al., 2013, p. 115).

In health policy, the explanatory power of policy transfer and diffusion models is tendentially rather limited (Starke & Tosun, 2019, p. 196). Following the argument of Makse and Volden (2011) that the characteristics of policies, particularly their combinability with prior practices and their complexity, influence whether they are diffused, it is not surprising that few policy diffusion studies focus on health policies. Finally, jurisdictions must also consider how policies will be implemented (Nicholson-Crotty & Carley, 2015). Given the often historically evolved and institutionally divergent structures of health care, diffusion in health policy is likely to occur only when institutions are newly established and given additional responsibilities, as in the case of evidence-based health agencies (Hassenteufel et al., 2017) or health technology assessment (HTA) (Löblová, 2016). In less federalized systems with shared responsibilities among health care organizations, subnational responsibilities can serve as opportunities for experimental evaluation of policy effectiveness (Volden, 2017). This research reemphasizes the need to consider institutional differences and predispositions in the study of health policy.

Moreover, the processes of harmonizing policies across Europe are less developed due to institutional challenges, and countries rarely want to transfer competences in this policy area to the supranational level (Martinsen et al., 2020). Consequently, internationalization, Europeanization, and diffusion models are expected to play a minor role in explaining health policy in France and Germany in recent decades.

However, even if limited, there is a certain international influence on national health policy programs. Joint membership in national or supranational bodies has been shown to drive the diffusion of policy knowledge so that, for example, changes in the hospital financing systems of a majority of OECD countries resulted in part from their positive effects on reducing health expenditures in other OECD countries (Gilardi et al., 2008, p. 568). Hassenteufel and Palier (2014) stress that the new economic and budgetary rules set by the European Union has increased the presence of deficit reduction instruments and arguments in the French political discourse. Although not yet driving French health policy reforms, the economic rules clearly put pressure on the national governments that hinders the adoption of rather leftist reforms involving an increased spending on health care and hazarding the consequences of augmented debt and deficit.

While the French health policy can be seen in part as a reaction to these international pressures, the neoliberal ideas put forward by Reagan and Thatcher translated into elements of competition prominently being introduced in Germany. These were borrowed from the experience of the Dutch reform in terms of regulated competition and the reference pricing system (Leiber et al., 2010), the US in terms of selective contracts (Cheng & Reinhardt, 2008), but not in France (Propper, 2018, p. 494), and Australia with regard to DRGs (Schreyögg et al., 2006). Although health care reforms in Germany strongly resembled the "Third Way" strategies as in the UK, one cannot speak of a true convergence of strategies and instruments, but rather of a similar way of legitimizing reforms (Bandelow, 2007b). Ultimately, the adoption of policy reforms from other countries depends heavily on existing institutions in the respective political systems and subsystems, especially in the health care sector, whose established structures make one-to-one policy transfer difficult (Verspohl, 2012, p. 308). Although the health care system in both France and Germany is based on a Bismarckian structure of contribution-financed SHI, and Bismarckian welfare states tend to converge (Hassenteufel & Palier, 2007), institutional differences regarding federalist, corporatist, and political structures make it difficult to copy many (at least structural) reforms.

While policy transfer and diffusion models obviously influenced the content of health care reforms in France and Germany, the question remains how the utilization of policy advice and scientific impulses are linked to biographies and thereby to actors' biographies. The endogenous role of scientific knowledge and advice in the policy process can help shed light on this. It is divided into two main strands of literature:

The first is concerned with evidence-based policymaking, more specifically how research is or should be formally embedded in the policy process and how the relationship between researchers and policy-makers is or should be (French, 2019). The use of experts and evidence in deliberative processes of citizen participation also fall under this conceptualization (Roberts et al., 2020), but are not considered in this contribution due to their marginal impact on policy processes. However, the involvement of expert advice in decision-making structures varies and depends on institutional structures such as cabinet decision-making and government composition (Fleischer, 2009). It can be achieved by taking into account suggestions and expertise from sectoral actors, such as interest groups. In the area of health policy, for example, medical and epidemiological advice could be relevant information for decisions regarding which services are reimbursed by sickness funds. However, evidence from other studies suggests that the consideration of interest groups on highly politicized issues depends less on their expertise than on their social support (Willems, 2020). More to the point, interest groups may even be disempowered if expert advice is used more intensively to inform and legitimize policy-making (Cross et al., 2021). Expert advice can also come from political parties or, in a supposedly neutral way, from the involvement of scientists in decision-making bodies or councils.

Under the label of evidence-based policy-making, some scholars now argue for systematic consideration of science by policy-makers. However, it is increasingly difficult to make evidence available to decision-makers in a productive way. Part of this challenge lies in science communication, as both the recipients of expert advice in policy are unclearly perceived and it is unclear exactly what is required of scientists to support decisions (Saretzki, 2019). One solution to this challenge may be ongoing exchanges between policy actors and experts, ideally in committees through which science is expected to have its greatest impact on policy (Bogenschneider & Bogenschneider, 2020; Peterson, 2018). Another challenge lies in the selection of expertise for policy decisions, also with regard to potential conflicts of interests, although McComas et al. (2005) note that experts in advisory bodies value expertise over impartiality. In German health policy, this challenge has been addressed by the largely impartial proposals developed in the SVR-G and the Enquete Commission (Knieps, 2009). However, greater collaboration between politics and science may also prove fruitful for coalition-building (Cairney et al., 2016, p. 401). Ensuring that scientific advice is considered over time requires long-term strategies and collaboration, a new form of co-production (Cairney & Oliver, 2017, p. 4).

This leads us to the second understanding of scientific knowledge and advice as a more group-centered perspective on advisory committees. In this regard, the literature on policy advice has revealed a large influence of advisors on policy-making processes. At the science-policy interface, Hoppe (2010) distinguishes several types of boundary workers that fill in diverse functions. The concept of policy advice is understood here less as scientific impulses for innovative policy ideas than as political advice. The closest to the notion of programmatic action is mega-policy strategy, as programmatic actors are focused on major changes and strategic outlooks (Hoppe, 2010). In fact, programmatic actors represent a specific type of science-policy relationship—they can be civil servants, policy advisors, or administrative actors of sectoral bodies who liaise with scientists and are informed by the evidence provided to develop new ideas and compile them into a strategic vision for the policy sector.

The institutions of expert advice involvement also vary depending on the political institutions surrounding them. In countries where political parties play a significant role in formulating policies, recruiting political elites, and preparing legislative proposals through parliamentary committees, party-affiliated foundations can have a considerable impact on the generation of ideas. Public administration research also suggests that the civil service tends to become politicized when it must provide expert advice with equal attention to political considerations (Craft & Howlett, 2017). However, Shaw and Eichbaum (2020) show that politicization of civil servants is not driven solely by exogenous factors, but is inherent in civil servants' sense of duty to their minister. They distinguish between different forms of politicization of the ministerial bureaucracy, focusing on the relationship between civil servants and political advisors and the extent to which political considerations moderate the provision of advice (Hustedt & Salomonsen, 2014, pp. 749-751). In partisan democracies, this is all the more relevant, because civil servants are selected in part on the basis of partisan ties and are thus prone to giving political rather than evidence-based advice.

On the other hand, expert advice may not only initiate new thinking, but also serve to confirm existing opinions or be instrumentalized in the struggle for "truth" (Kisby, 2010). Heikkila et al. (2020) show that scientific information almost always leads policy actors to corroborate their preferences and that this can only be broken if actor networks are diversified, actors are familiarized with science, or scientific knowledge is coupled with existing risk perceptions. Thus, for science to generate new policy ideas, actors must be brought together who ideally do not have preexisting policy preferences. This is even easier in policy sectors that have not yet been touched, although examples of French and German health policy show that this is possible even in highly contested policy sectors blocked by vested interests, as long as scientific uncertainty does not prevail and prevent far-reaching legislation (Bromley-Trujillo & Karch, 2019), and as long as the actors initiating change do not belong to these competing coalitions. As a consequence, the following hypothesis is postulated that sees the institutionalization of advice and ideas as a potential necessary condition for programmatic action.

Science Policy Hypothesis
Enabling the inclusion and institutionalization of scientific advice is a necessary condition for the generation of innovative ideas and inspires policy programs in the policy process. Such venues of intellectual reflection and discussion are necessary also to inform and support the formation of programmatic groups and successful programmatic action.

Taking the institutionalization of expert advice as a necessary institutional condition for programmatic action, it is interesting to see how this is shaped in different institutional settings. There are different forms and dimension of advice. A prominent view in public administration is on ministerial advisors, who are assigned to a single minister and are functionally equivalent across countries, acting between politics and bureaucracy (Hustedt et al., 2017). An example are the ministerial cabinets in France (De Lamothe, 1965) or Italy, where career patterns lead to links between sectoral experts in the ministerial bureaucracy and other sectoral bodies (Di Mascio & Natalini, 2013, p. 338). The empirical study has shown that these ministerial cabinets are also highly relevant for programmatic action. Their members have been trained (which is a link to the institution of elite formation) to provide expertise, and the networks they form influence policy-making and perpetuate themselves (Rouban, 2007, p. 492).

Although particular to the French political system, the functional equivalent found in other countries is the extent to which new ideas are formulated and driven by a group of actors close to the state apparatus (such as the minister). Thus, it is not ministerial cabinets per se that enable programmatic action, but the institutionalization of expert advice at a particular point in the policy process within groups that subsequently advance their jointly developed ideas. This mainly works through the formation of shared biographical trajectories through these expert bodies. In line with the literature on policy transfer and diffusion, it must be noted that these biographies can also be driven internationally.

3.5   INTERMEDIARY CONCLUSION: INSTITUTIONAL CONDITIONS FOR PROGRAMMATIC ACTION

The review of the literature strands outlined above served two purposes: First, to highlight the gap that the PAF fills as an additional lens on policy processes by identifying the distinctive features of existing theoretical frameworks and situating the PAF within these lines of research. Since these perspectives may also offer alternative explanations for the policies explained in the empirical analysis using the PAF, it is important to clarify in which situations these theoretical perspectives prove particularly useful—and in which they do not—which will be an important argument for the usefulness of the PAF in unfolding explanatory power. The extent to which they can serve as alternative explanations for the observed policy changes will be addressed later. The second goal was to use existing research on political institutions and public policy and in particular the ways in which institutions are incorporated in theoretical mechanisms explaining policy processes, to theorize the opportunities and constraints of programmatic action. If one pursues the goal of the PAF to be applicable and insightful across different political systems, it is imperative to work out the extent to which country-specific and comparative studies of the institutional settings within which policy-making takes place can help sharpen the PAF concepts and identify the relevant institutions for programmatic action. In this regard, it is particularly fruitful to incorporate the insights of established institutional analyses in explaining group formation and the emergence of ideas as well as their subsequent success. Indeed, the theoretical perspectives presented offer points of departure for PAF to develop theoretical arguments, particularly regarding the ways in which institutions may influence programmatic group formation and the success of programmatic groups and policy programs. While such an overview provides a starting point, only later empirical investigation will reveal which institutions have proven relevant to programmatic action.

To bring clarity and order back into the previously extensively discussed theoretical jungle, this chapter briefly summarizes the core explanation for policy change advocated by theoretical perspectives and justifies why and which elements of the PAF present add value to the theoretical state of the art. While some institutionalist arguments of existing theories also appear transferable to the PAF, such as corporatist and decentralized structures, the later analysis will also add undiscovered institutional drivers of programmatic action, which include institutional change in addition to institutions promoting elite formation and innovation of ideas.

Table 3.1 provides an overview of policy process frameworks, their foundations, core explanation, and understanding and relevance of institutions. The postulated hypotheses assume that these institutions observed in other theoretical perspectives are potentially also relevant to the PAF or, more specifically, to programmatic group formation and the success of programmatic groups and policy programs. However, the postulated hypotheses point toward a great importance of education and systems of elite formation, as well as of the institutionalization of policy advice, to programmatic action.

The core explanations for policy change vary depending on the theoretical perspectives: Policy change in response to problem pressures, external events, or situational factors such as opening policy windows represent the perspectives adopted by the MSF, which further specify the institutional conditions under which policy entrepreneurs are likely to succeed in their attempt to push through their policy proposal. Long-term processes of policy change, on the other hand, tend to be represented by network theories and the ACF, which propose to conceptualize policy change as a process that takes place over a decade or more. The PAF brings to this set of theoretical perspectives a view of shared biographies and resulting collaborations based on a policy program to include policy change over at least a decade to a generation of programmatic actors (30 years or more).

Table 3.1 Overview on scope of theories of policy change and stability

Theoretical perspectives	Micro-level foundation	Core explanation for policy change	Relevance of institutions prominently discussed in comparative politics
Advocacy Coalition Framework (ACF)	Belief systems and biased perception	Internal shocks, external events, negotiated agreements, learning	Constitutional rules and the political system shape opportunity structures for coalitions
Multiple Streams Framework (MSF)	Ambiguity and bounded rationality due to uncertainty and time constraints	Policy entrepreneurs, windows of opportunity, coupling of streams	Institutions (structures, resources, culture of policy sector) shape actions and strategies available to policy entrepreneurs/ institutional entrepreneurship
Network Theories	Bounded rationality or rational-strategic thinking	Collaboration of policy actors on the basis of trust, knowledge, experience, issues	Institutions foster networks, opportunities, and occasions to create networks, trust through institutions
Programmatic Action Framework (PAF)	Identification with social groups, search for authority	Programmatic groups and policy programs	Success of programmatic groups depends on whether they involve corporatist and/or subnational actors and use corporatist and/or decentralized structures to promote their program

Source: Own compilation

The key innovation, then, is that it assumes career policy actors seeking greater authority in the state and that it assumes that these actors form programmatic groups based on shared experiences and pursue a policy program of their ideas to achieve their goals.

Under what institutional conditions both the formation of programmatic groups and the success of programmatic groups and their policy programs is achieved is the core question of this book. After looking at existing research on the interplay of actors and institutions in policy processes, it is possible to assess which institutions are potentially relevant for the course of programmatic action. This assessment is based on the previously elaborated Programmatic Action Framework. Table 3.1 therefore contains a column outlining the institutions taken from existing theoretical approaches and the ways in which they might influence the formation and success of programmatic groups. In the following paragraphs, this relationship is exemplified for each theoretical strand.

Two frequently addressed institutions in comparative politics that have an influence on policy-making and actors are corporatism and federalism. Corporatist structures can generally be seen as a facilitating factor for group formation. Their institutionalized venues for policy-making offer numerous opportunities for exchange and cooperation. Programmatic groups have a chance of success with their programs if they succeed in making strategic use of these corporatist structures and integrating the corporatist actors into their programmatic group. The same is true for varying levels of federalism. Subnational structures generally support the formation of groups and exchange among policy actors and therefore are necessary to include when programmatic groups seek success because they are relevant in policy-making processes.

External events, socioeconomic developments, and public crises are often integrated into policy process frameworks (as external shocks in the ACF or focusing events in the MSF) and thus always represent catalysts of processes, be it group formation or policy success (Saurugger & Terpan, 2016). Therefore, with respect to the PAF, it is equally reasonable to assume that these situational conditions act as accelerators of group formation and also represent opportunities for short-term ad hoc cooperation. Moreover, they can be useful and contribute to programmatic success if programmatic groups use these problem pressures and crises to advance their own policy program, and if the policy program is able and flexible enough to react to these developments and provide an adequate response to the emerging problems.

In actor-centered approaches to policy processes, namely MSF, ACF, and network theories, the relevant institutions are always those that provide resources to actors or opportunities for actors to behave in ways that favor policy change. These include some of the institutions of veto players, federalism, corporatism, parties, and path dependencies mentioned above. Network theories in particular emphasize the role that institutional opportunities play in cooperation and collective action. In sum, institutional opportunities that promote networking among policy actors and those that provide policy actors with the resources and strategies necessary to pursue their goals contribute to programmatic group formation. The subsequent success of these strategies then depends, in turn, on whether programmatic groups have the necessary resources to achieve their goals in the institutional settings and whether they use a coherent narrative that fits their strategy.

When talking about institutions, policy process frameworks basically mean the same type of political institutions introduced by prominent typologies such as those of Lijphart (2012), Tsebelis, or Hall and Soskice (2001). These are used in analyses that apply the PET (Fernández-i-Marín et al., 2019, p. 14; Kuhlmann & van der Heijden, 2018, p. 329), theories of coalition formation (Fischer, 2015, p. 246), and the MSF (Zohlnhöfer et al., 2016).

While Table 3.1 already contains an assessment of the potential relevance of political institutions for the PAF, formulating concrete expectations about the (directional) impact of well-known and widely recognized institutional settings on programmatic action seems less straightforward. In particular, this is because institutional conditions exert a different influence on programmatic action depending on whether the emerging programmatic group under analysis already occupies key positions in the policy sector (yes/no) and whether it faces an established programmatic group that already holds key positions (yes/no). It follows that institutional differences per country do not necessarily explain programmatic group formation and programmatic success, or at least have different effects depending on the characteristics and situation of the programmatic group. To illustrate the impact of each institutional factor on the different stages a programmatic group may be in Fig. 3.1 shows a coordinate system listing institutional influences on opportunities and constraints for programmatic group formation and programmatic group and policy program success, depending on whether it is an emerging programmatic group with or without key positions filled. Furthermore, the effects of institutions are visualized in cases where the emerging programmatic group faces an established programmatic group with or without key positions occupied. The chances for group formation and programmatic success are always evaluated for an emerging programmatic group.

Depending on the characteristics and situation of an emerging programmatic group, how would institutions affect the formation of the programmatic group and its subsequent success? Four scenarios are conceivable here:

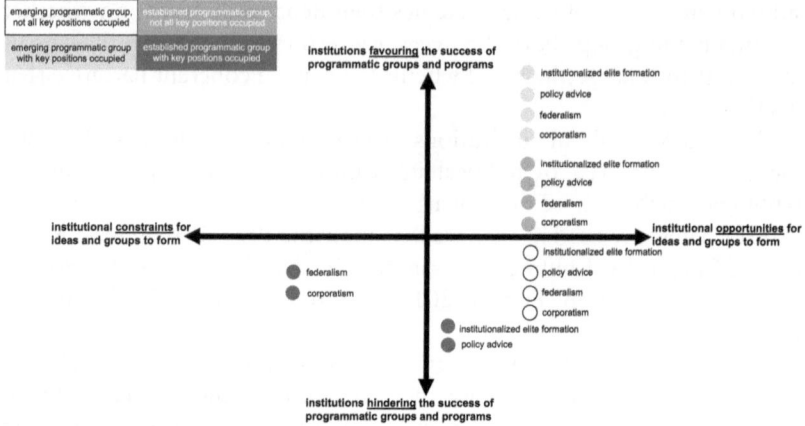

Fig. 3.1 Institutional opportunities and constraints for programmatic action. Source: Own compilation

Emerging Programmatic Group, Not All Key Positions Occupied

Imagine many policy actors who are potential programmatic actors. This group of actors does not (yet) occupy all the necessary positions that would allow them to participate directly in all the arenas where policy ideas are debated, and decisions are made. In such cases, the degree to which group-forming institutions are institutionalized with the participation of relevant actors will contribute significantly to whether a programmatic group will form and succeed, because the group needs this kind of connection to gain the positions necessary to possess resources for success. Decentralized structures in weak federalism and corporatism provide a variety of opportunities and venues to connect and form groups. Given the decentralized or corporatist structures that the programmatic group then penetrates and given that the group then includes members across these structures, its resources increase and its success solidifies. Other networking opportunities and institutionalized biographical paths are even more conducive to interaction among policy actors, especially when no established programmatic group dominates such venues. However, in this case, the subsequent chances of success are not as good as those promised by corporatist or decentralized structures in the short term. Since networking events offer many points of contact, a programmatic group can also be attacked more easily. For an emerging programmatic group that does not occupy key positions, the necessary resources to adopt and implement its program are lacking. Accordingly, neither the formation nor the success of programmatic groups is expected.

Emerging Programmatic Group, with Key Positions Occupied

However, when considering an emerging programmatic group that already occupies central key positions, several institutions favor its formation and subsequent success. Federalism and corporatism, as well as institutionalized education systems and policy advice, favor the emergence of ideas and groups because they provide a pool of policy actors among whom are already actors in the necessary positions that can influence policy-making at many levels. Consequently, this favors both the formation and the subsequent success of programmatic groups because they benefit from multiple opportunities to collaborate, include all relevant actors in their group and program, and engage in intellectual discussion that they control through key positions.

Established Programmatic Group, Not All Key Positions Occupied

When the emerging programmatic group faces an already established programmatic group, the question of group formation and success depends on which key positions are still held by the established programmatic group. If it has already lost key positions, this provides some opportunities for the emerging programmatic group. Again, federalism and corporatism, as well as institutions that foster group formation through institutionalized career paths and advisory systems, favor group formation and provide an anchor for the emerging programmatic group to challenge the established programmatic group. If they can engage policy actors in the key positions not held by the existing dominant programmatic group in an inclusive policy program, this favors their success.

Established Programmatic Group, with Key Positions Occupied

Finally, the most uncomfortable situation for an emerging programmatic group is when there is an established programmatic group that occupies all the key positions. As Bandelow and Hornung (2020) show, this is the moment when the incumbent programmatic group will be strongest. Since all key positions are occupied by the dominant programmatic group, all institutions are under its control and thus the stabilizing institutions play into its hands. Federalist and corporatist structures are shaped by the policy program. Only the opportunities for networking and collaborative forums through elite formation and expert advice remain, offering the potential for programmatic groups to form, but they will not be successful because key positions belong to the established programmatic group. In such cases, policy actors might simply join the dominant programmatic group to pursue their goals, comparable to what is called engaging in mainstream politics in party politics (Schumacher & van Kersbergen, 2014).

What is also apparent from this coordinate system is that the institutional factors can be found in the upper right or lower left quadrant in each case. This means that the questions about the formation of programmatic groups and their success are theoretically (and possibly also empirically) very closely linked. Accordingly, the expected influence of institutions equally regards the formation and success of groups.

Summarizing the results of these theoretical considerations, it is clear that the effects of the institutions examined here on programmatic action are complex and also depend on the stage a programmatic group is at, at any given time. While some political institutions can shed light on one or another aspect of favorable circumstances for programmatic group formation and programmatic success, the institutions of programmatic action appear to have a different focus than the previously known and used in comparative politics and policy process research, namely a focus on the formation of groups and the involvement of innovative ideas for programs to be successful.

References

Andersen, S. C., & Jakobsen, M. L. (2018). Political Pressure, Conformity Pressure, and Performance Information as Drivers of Public Sector Innovation Adoption. *International Public Management Journal, 21*(2), 213–242. https://doi.org/10.1080/10967494.2018.1425227

Andrews, J. T., & Montinola, G. R. (2004). Veto Players and the Rule of Law in Emerging Democracies. *Comparative Political Studies, 37*(1), 55–87. https://doi.org/10.1177/0010414003260125

Angelova, M., Bäck, H., Müller, W. C., & Strobl, D. (2018). Veto Player Theory and Reform Making in Western Europe. *European Journal of Political Research, 57*(2), 282–307. https://doi.org/10.1111/1475-6765.12226

Auel, K. (2014). Intergovernmental Relations in German Federalism: Cooperative Federalism, Party Politics and Territorial Conflicts. *Comparative European Politics, 12*(4), 422–443. https://doi.org/10.1057/cep.2014.13

Baccaro, L. (2003). What is Alive and What is Dead in the Theory of Corporatism. *British Journal of Industrial Relations, 41*(4), 683–706. https://doi.org/10.1046/j.1467-8543.2003.00294.x

Bach, T., & Veit, S. (2018). The Determinants of Promotion to High Public Office in Germany: Partisan Loyalty, Political Craft, or Managerial Competencies? *Journal of Public Administration Research and Theory, 28*(2), 254–269. https://doi.org/10.1093/jopart/mux041

Bailey, M. A., Rom, M. C., & Taylor, M. M. (2004). State Competition in Higher Education: A Race to the Top, or a Race to the Bottom? *Economics of Governance, 5*(1), 53–75. https://doi.org/10.1007/s10101-002-0052-0

Bandelow, N. C. (1998). *Gesundheitspolitik: Der Staat in der Hand einzelner Interessengruppen? Probleme, Erklärungen, Reformen.* Springer VS (Leske + Budrich).

Bandelow, N. C. (2007a). Ärzteverbände. Niedergang eines Erfolgsmodells? In T. von Winter & U. Willems (Eds.), *Interessenverbände in Deutschland* (pp. 271–293). VS Verlag für Sozialwissenschaften.

Bandelow, N. C. (2007b). Der Dritte Weg in der britischen und deutschen Gesundheitspolitik: Separate Reformpfade trotz ideologischer Nähe? *Zeitschrift für Sozialreform, 53*(2), 127–145.

Bandelow, N. C., & Hornung, J. (2020). Policy Programme Cycles Through Old and New Programmatic Groups. *Journal of Public Policy, early view.* doi:https://doi.org/10.1017/S0143814X20000185

Bastiaens, I., & Postnikov, E. (2017). Greening Up: The Effects of Environmental Standards in EU and US Trade Agreements. *Environmental Politics, 26*(5), 847–869. https://doi.org/10.1080/09644016.2017.1338213

Baumgartner, F. R., Brouard, S., Grossman, E., Lazardeux, S. G., & Moody, J. (2014). Divided Government, Legislative Productivity, and Policy Change in the USA and France. *Governance, 27*(3), 423–447. https://doi.org/10.1111/gove.12047

Baybeck, B., Berry, W. D., & Siegel, D. A. (2011). A Strategic Theory of Policy Diffusion via Intergovernmental Competition. *The Journal of Politics, 73*(1), 232–247. https://doi.org/10.1017/S0022381610000988

Becher, M., & Brouard, S. (2020). Executive Accountability Beyond Outcomes: Experimental Evidence on Public Evaluations of Powerful Prime Ministers. *American Journal of Political Science, n/a*(n/a). doi:https://doi.org/10.1111/ajps.12558

Bernardi, L., Bischof, D., & Wouters, R. (2020). The Public, the Protester, and the Bill: Do Legislative Agendas Respond to Public Opinion Signals? *Journal of European Public Policy, 1*, 22. https://doi.org/10.1080/13501763.2020.1729226

Berry, F. S., & Berry, W. D. (2017). Innovation and Diffusion Models in Policy Research. In C. M. Weible & P. A. Sabatier (Eds.), *Theories of the Policy Process* (4th ed., pp. 253–300). Westview Press.

Best, H., & Higley, J. (2018). *The Palgrave Handbook of Political Elites*. Macmillan Publishers Ltd.

Bezes, P., & Le Lidec, P. (2015). The French Politics of Retrenchment (2007–2012): Institutions and Blame Avoidance Strategies. *International Review of Administrative Sciences, 81*(3), 498–521. https://doi.org/10.1177/0020852315576712

Blondel, J., & Müller-Rommel, F. (2007). Political Elites. In R. J. Dalton & H.-D. Klingemann (Eds.), *The Oxford Handbook of Political Behavior*. Oxford University Press.

Bogenschneider, K., & Bogenschneider, B. N. (2020). Empirical Evidence from State Legislators: How, When, and Who Uses Research. *Psychology, Public Policy, and Law, 26*(4), 413–424. https://doi.org/10.1037/law0000232

Bräuninger, T., Debus, M., Müller, J., & Stecker, C. (2019). Party Competition and Government Formation in Germany: Business as Usual or New Patterns? *German Politics, 28*(1), 80–100. https://doi.org/10.1080/09644008.2018.1538362

Breunig, C. (2014). Content and Dynamics of Legislative Agendas in Germany. In C. Green-Pedersen & S. Walgrave (Eds.), *Agenda Setting, Policies, and Political Systems: A Comparative Approach* (pp. 125–144). University of Chicago Press.

Bromley-Trujillo, R., & Karch, A. (2019). Salience, Scientific Uncertainty, and the Agenda-Setting Power of Science. *Policy Studies Journal, n/a*(n/a). doi:https://doi.org/10.1111/psj.12373

Brouard, S. (2009). The Politics of Constitutional Veto in France: Constitutional Council, Legislative Majority and Electoral Competition. *West European Politics, 32*(2), 384–403. https://doi.org/10.1080/01402380802670719

Brouard, S., & Hönnige, C. (2017). Constitutional Courts as Veto Players: Lessons From the United States, France and Germany. *European Journal of Political Research, 56*(3), 529–552. https://doi.org/10.1111/1475-6765.12192

Brunner, M., & Debus, M. (2008). Between Programmatic Interests and Party Politics: The German Bundesrat in the Legislative Process. *German Politics, 17*(3), 232–251. https://doi.org/10.1080/09644000802300288

Burge, G. S., & Rogers, C. L. (2016). Leaders, Followers, and Asymmetric Local Tax Policy Diffusion. *Journal of Regional Science, 56*(2), 313–331. https://doi.org/10.1111/jors.12242

Busch, P. O., & Jörgens, H. (2005). The International Sources of Policy Convergence: Explaining the Spread of Environmental Policy Innovations. *Journal of European Public Policy, 12*(5), 860–884. https://doi.org/10.1080/13501760500161514

Busch, P.-O., Jörgens, H., & Tews, K. (2005). The Global Diffusion of Regulatory Instruments: The Making of a New International Environmental Regime. *The ANNALS of the American Academy of Political and Social Science, 598*(1), 146–167. https://doi.org/10.1177/0002716204272355

Butler, D. M., Volden, C., Dynes, A. M., & Shor, B. (2017). Ideology, Learning, and Policy Diffusion: Experimental Evidence. *American Journal of Political Science, 61*(1), 37–49. https://doi.org/10.1111/ajps.12213

Cairney, P., & Oliver, K. (2017). Evidence-based Policymaking is not like Evidence-based Medicine, So How Far Should You Go to Bridge the Divide Between Evidence and Policy? *Health Research Policy and Systems, 15*(35), 1–11.

Cairney, P., Oliver, K., & Wellstead, A. (2016). To Bridge the Divide between Evidence and Policy: Reduce Ambiguity as Much as Uncertainty. *Public Administration Review, 76*(3), 399–402. https://doi.org/10.1111/puar.12555

Capano, G. (2018). Reconceptualizing Layering—From Mode of Institutional Change to Mode of Institutional Design: Types and Outputs. *Public Administration, 1*, 1. https://doi.org/10.1111/padm.12583

Cawson, A. (1985). *Organized Interests and the State: Studies in Meso-Corporatism.* SAGE Publications Ltd..

Chamorel, P. (2019). Macron Versus the Yellow Vests. *Journal of Democracy, 30*(4), 48–62. https://doi.org/10.1353/jod.2019.0068

Cheibub, J. A., Elkins, Z., & Ginsburg, T. (2014). Beyond Presidentialism and Parliamentarism. *British Journal of Political Science, 44*(3), 515–544. https://doi.org/10.1017/S000712341300032X

Cheng, T.-M., & Reinhardt, U. E. (2008). Shepherding Major Health System Reforms: A Conversation With German Health Minister Ulla Schmidt. *Health Affairs, 27*(Suppl. 1), w204–w213. https://doi.org/10.1377/hlthaff.27.3.w204

Cole, A. (1993). The Presidential Party and the Fifth Republic. *West European Politics, 16*(2), 49–66. https://doi.org/10.1080/01402389308424960

Cox, A. (1981). Corporatism as Reductionism: the Analytic Limits of the Corporatist Thesis. *Government and Opposition, 16*(1), 78–95. https://doi.org/10.1111/j.1477-7053.1981.tb00301.x

Craft, J., & Howlett, M. (2017). The Dual Dynamics of Policy Advisory Systems: The Impact of Externalization and Politicization on Policy Advice. *Policy and Society, 32*(3), 187–197. https://doi.org/10.1016/j.polsoc.2013.07.001

Cross, J. P., Eising, R., Hermansson, H., & Spohr, F. (2021). Business Interests, Public Interests, and Experts in Parliamentary Committees: their Impact on Legislative Amendments in the German Bundestag. *West European Politics, 44*(2), 354–377. https://doi.org/10.1080/01402382.2019.1672025

Czada, R. (2015). "Post-Democracy" and the Public Sphere: Informality and Transparency in Negotiated Decision-Making. In V. Schneider & B. Eberlein (Eds.), *Complex Democracy: Varieties, Crises, and Transformations* (pp. 231–246). Springer International Publishing.

Dahl, R. A. (1961). *Who Governs? Democracy and Power in an American City*. Yale University Press.

De Lamothe, A. D. (1965). Ministerial Cabinets in France. *Public Administration, 43*(4), 365–379. https://doi.org/10.1111/j.1467-9299.1965.tb01658.x

Debus, M., & Bräuninger, T. (2008). Intra-Party Factions and Coalition Bargaining in Germany. In D. Giannetti & K. Benoit (Eds.), *Intra-Party Politics and Coalition Governments in Parliamentary Democracies* (pp. 121–145). Routledge.

Dent, M., Howorth, C., Mueller, F., & Preuschoft, C. (2004). Archetype Transition in the German Health Service? The Attempted Modernization of Hospitals in a North German State. *Public Administration, 82*(3), 727–742. https://doi.org/10.1111/j.0033-3298.2004.00416.x

Derlien, H.-U. (1991). Historical Legacy and Recent Developments in the German Higher Civil Service. *International Review of Administrative Sciences, 57*(3), 385–401. https://doi.org/10.1177/002085239105700306

Di Mascio, F., & Natalini, A. (2013). Analysing the Role of Ministerial Cabinets in Italy: Legacy and Temporality in the Study of Administrative Reforms. *International Review of Administrative Sciences, 79*(2), 328–346. https://doi.org/10.1177/0020852313477972

Elgie, R. (2009). Duverger, Semi-presidentialism and the Supposed French Archetype. *West European Politics, 32*(2), 248–267. https://doi.org/10.1080/01402380802670453

Engler, F., & Dümig, K. (2017). Political Parties and MPs' Morality Policy Voting Behaviour: Evidence from Germany. *Parliamentary Affairs, 70*(3), 548–568. https://doi.org/10.1093/pa/gsw034

Eppner, S., & Ganghof, S. (2017). Institutional Veto Players and Cabinet Formation: The Veto Control Hypothesis Reconsidered. *European Journal of Political Research, 56*(1), 169–186. https://doi.org/10.1111/1475-6765.12172

Fasone, C. (2017). The Influence of Standing Committees on the Forms of Government. The Case of France, Italy, and the UK. *Rivista Di Diritti Comparati, 1*(1), 15–54.

Fernández-i-Marín, X., Hurka, S., Knill, C., & Steinebach, Y. (2019). Systemic Dynamics of Policy Change: Overcoming Some Blind Spots of Punctuated Equilibrium Theory. *Policy Studies Journal, n/a*(n/a). doi:https://doi.org/10.1111/psj.12379

Fischer, M. (2015). Institutions and Coalitions in Policy Processes: a Cross-sectoral Comparison. *Journal of Public Policy, 35*(2), 245–268. https://doi.org/10.1017/S0143814X14000166

Fleischer, J. (2009). Power Resources of Parliamentary Executives: Policy Advice in the UK and Germany. *West European Politics, 32*(1), 196–214. https://doi.org/10.1080/01402380802509941

François, B. (1997). Le Conseil Constitutionnel et la Cinquième République: Réflexions sur l'Émergence et les Effets du Contrôle de Constitutionnalité en France. *Revue française de science politique, 47*(3/4), 377–403. Retrieved from http://www.jstor.org/stable/43121805

French, R. D. (2019). Is it Time to Give Up on Evidence-Based Policy? Four Answers. *Policy & Politics, 47*(1), 151–168.

Ganghof, S., & Bräuninger, T. (2006). Government Status and Legislative Behaviour: Partisan Veto Players in Australia, Denmark, Finland and Germany. *Party Politics, 12*(4), 521–539. https://doi.org/10.1177/1354068806064732

Genieys, W., & Hassenteufel, P. (2012). Comprendre le changement dans les politiques publiques ? L'approche programmatique. Retrieved from https://hal.archives-ouvertes.fr/hal-01401805

Genieys, W., & Smyrl, M. (2008). Inside the Autonomous State: Programmatic Elites in the Reform of French Health Policy. *Governance, 21*(1), 75–93. https://doi.org/10.1111/j.1468-0491.2007.00386.x

Gerlinger, T. (2010). Health Care Reform in Germany. *German Policy Studies, 6*(1), 107–142.

Giaimo, S. (1995). Health Care Reform in Britain and Germany: Recasting the Political Bargain with the Medical Profession. *Governance, 8*(3), 354–379. https://doi.org/10.1111/j.1468-0491.1995.tb00215.x

Giaimo, S., & Manow, P. (1999). Adapting the Welfare State: The Case of Health Care Reform in Britain, Germany, and the United States. *Comparative Political Studies, 32*(8), 967–1000. https://doi.org/10.1177/0010414099032008003

Gilardi, F., Füglister, K., & Luyet, S. (2008). Learning From Others: The Diffusion of Hospital Financing Reforms in OECD Countries. *Comparative Political Studies, 42*(4), 549–573. https://doi.org/10.1177/0010414008327428

Giuliani, M. (2016). Patterns of Democracy Reconsidered: The Ambiguous Relationship Between Corporatism and Consensualism. *European Journal of Political Research, 55*(1), 22–42. https://doi.org/10.1111/1475-6765.12117

Godbout, J.-F., & Foucault, M. (2013). French Legislative Voting in the Fifth Republic. *French Politics, 11*(4), 307–331. https://doi.org/10.1057/fp.2013.17

Godt, P. J. (1987). Confrontation, Consent, and Corporatism: State Strategies and the Medical Profession in France, Great Britain, and West Germany. *Journal of Health Politics, Policy and Law, 12*(3), 459–480. https://doi.org/10.1215/03616878-12-3-459

Gross, M., & Krauss, S. (2019). Topic Coverage of Coalition Agreements in Multi-Level Settings: The Case of Germany. *German Politics, 1*, 22. https://doi.org/10.1080/09644008.2019.1658077

Grossback, L. J., Nicholson-Crotty, S., & Peterson, D. A. M. (2004). Ideology and Learning in Policy Diffusion. *American Politics Research, 32*(5), 521–545. https://doi.org/10.1177/1532673X04263801

Grossman, E. (2009). The President's Choice? Government and Cabinet Turnover under the Fifth Republic. *West European Politics, 32*(2), 268–286. https://doi.org/10.1080/01402380802670545

Grossman, E., & Sauger, N. (2009). The End of Ambiguity? Presidents versus Parties or the Four Phases of the Fifth Republic. *West European Politics, 32*(2), 423–437. https://doi.org/10.1080/01402380802670743

Ha, E. (2007). Globalization, Veto Players, and Welfare Spending. *Comparative Political Studies, 41*(6), 783–813. https://doi.org/10.1177/0010414006298938

Hacker, J. S. (2004). Review Article: Dismantling the Health Care State? Political Institutions, Public Policies and the Comparative Politics of Health Reform. *British Journal of Political Science, 34*(4), 693–724. https://doi.org/10.1017/S0007123404000250

Hager, C., & Hamagami, N. (2020). Local Renewable Energy Initiatives in Germany and Japan in a Changing National Policy Environment. *Review of Policy Research, n/a*(n/a). doi:https://doi.org/10.1111/ropr.12372

Hall, P. A., & Soskice, D. (Eds.). (2001). *Varieties of Capitalism: The Institutional Foundations of Comparative Advantage.* Oxford Univ. Press.

Hallerberg, M. (2011). Empirical Applications of Veto Player Analysis and Institutional Effectiveness. In T. König, M. Debus, & G. Tsebelis (Eds.), *Reform Processes and Policy Change: Veto Players and Decision-Making in Modern Democracies* (pp. 21–42). Springer.

Hassenteufel, P. (1996). The Medical Profession and Health Insurance Policies: A Franco-German Comparison. *Journal of European Public Policy, 3*(3), 461–480. https://doi.org/10.1080/13501769608407044

Hassenteufel, P. (1997). *Les médecins face à l'Etat: Une comparaison européenne.* Presses de la Fondation nationale des sciences politiques.

Hassenteufel, P., Benamouzig, D., Minonzio, J., & Robelet, M. (2017). Policy Diffusion and Translation: The Case of Evidence-based Health Agencies in Europe. *Novos estudos CEBRAP, 36,* 77–96.

Hassenteufel, P., & Palier, B. (2007). Towards Neo-Bismarckian Health Care States?: Comparing Health Insurance Reforms in Bismarckian Welfare Systems. *Social Policy & Administration, 41*(6), 574–596. https://doi.org/10.1111/j.1467-9515.2007.00573.x

Hassenteufel, P., & Palier, B. (2014). Still the Sound of Silence? Towards a New Phase in the Europeanisation of Welfare State Policies in France. *Comparative European Politics, 13*(1), 112–130. https://doi.org/10.1057/cep.2014.44

Hassenteufel, P., Schweyer, F.-X., Gerlinger, T., Henkel, R., Lückenbach, C., & Reiter, R. (2020). The Role of Professional Groups in Policy Change: Physician's Organizations and the Issue of Local Medical Provision Shortages in France and Germany. *European Policy Analysis, 6*(1), 38–57. https://doi.org/10.1002/epa2.1073

Hayward, J. (2004). Parliament and the French Government's Domination of the Legislative Process. *The Journal of Legislative Studies, 10*(2-3), 79–97. https://doi.org/10.1080/1357233042000322238

Heikkila, T., Weible, C., & Gerlak, A. K. (2020). When Does Science Persuade (or Not Persuade) in High Conflict Policy Contexts? *Public Administration, n/a*(n/a). doi:https://doi.org/10.1111/padm.12655

Heinze, R. G., & Schmid, J. (1997). Industrial Change and Meso-corporatism — A Comparative View on Three German States. *European Planning Studies, 5*(5), 597–617. https://doi.org/10.1080/09654319708720421

Hoffmann-Lange, U. (2007). Methods of Elite Research. In R. J. Dalton & H.-D. Klingemann (Eds.), *The Oxford Handbook of Political Behavior* (pp. 910–928). Oxford University Press.

Hohendorf, L., Saalfeld, T., & Sieberer, U. (2020). Veto Power Fosters Cooperative Behaviour: Institutional Incentives and Government-opposition Voting in the German Bundestag. *West European Politics, 1*, 25. https://doi.org/10.1080/01402382.2020.1739868

Hoppe, R. (2010). From "Knowledge Use" Towards "Boundary Work": Sketch of an Emerging New Agenda for Inquiry Into Science-policy Interaction. In R. J. in 't Veld (Ed.), *Knowledge Democracy: Consequences for Science, Politics, and Media* (pp. 169–186). Springer Berlin Heidelberg.

Hornung, J., Rüsenberg, R., Eckert, F., & Bandelow, N. C. (2020). New Insights into Coalition Negotiations – The Case of German Government Formation. *Negotiation Journal, 36*, 331–352. https://doi.org/10.1111/nejo.12310

Hustedt, T., Kolltveit, K., & Salomonsen, H. H. (2017). Ministerial Advisers in Executive Government: Out From the Dark and Into the Limelight. *Public Administration, 95*(2), 299–311. https://doi.org/10.1111/padm.12329

Hustedt, T., & Salomonsen, H. H. (2014). Ensuring Political Responsiveness: Politicization Mechanisms in Ministerial Bureaucracies. *International Review of Administrative Sciences, 80*(4), 746–765. https://doi.org/10.1177/0020852314533449

Immergut, E. M. (1990). Institutions, Veto Points, and Policy Results: A Comparative Analysis of Health Care. *Journal of Public Policy, 10*(4), 391–416. https://doi.org/10.1017/S0143814X00006061

Immergut, E. M. (2006). Institutional Constraints on Policy. In M. Moran, M. Rein, & R. Goodin (Eds.), *The Oxford Handbook of Public Policy* (pp. 557–572). Oxford University Press.

Jensen, C., & Wenzelburger, G. (2020). New Evidence on the Effect of Partisanship on the Welfare State. In R. Careja, P. Emmenegger, & N. Giger (Eds.), *The European Social Model under Pressure: Liber Amicorum in Honour of Klaus Armingeon* (pp. 123–137). Springer Fachmedien Wiesbaden.

Jensen, J. L. (2003). Policy Diffusion through Institutional Legitimation: State Lotteries. *Journal of Public Administration Research and Theory, 13*(4), 521–541. https://doi.org/10.1093/jpart/mug033

Johnson, C., & Tonkiss, F. (2002). The Third Influence: the Blair Government and Australian Labor. *Policy & Politics, 30*(1), 5–18.

Keeler, J. T. S. (1993). Executive Power and Policy-making Patterns in France: Gauging the Impact of Fifth Republic Institutions. *West European Politics, 16*(4), 518–544. https://doi.org/10.1080/01402389308424989

Keman, H., & Pennings, P. (1995). Managing Political and Societal Conflict in Democracies: Do Consensus and Corporatism Matter? *British Journal of Political Science, 25*(2), 271–281. https://doi.org/10.1017/S000712340 0007183

Kerrouche, E. (2006). The French Assemblée Nationale: The Case of a Weak Legislature? *The Journal of Legislative Studies, 12*(3-4), 336–365. https://doi.org/10.1080/13572330500483930

Kisby, B. (2010). Interpreting Facts, Verifying Interpretations: Public Policy, Truth and Evidence. *Public Policy and Administration, 26*(1), 107–127. https://doi.org/10.1177/0952076710375784

Klenk, T. (2018). Interessenlagen und Interessenpolitik im Gesundheitssektor. In T. Spier & C. Strünck (Eds.), *Ärzteverbände und ihre Mitglieder: Zwischen Einfluss- und Mitgliederlogik* (pp. 19–46). Springer Fachmedien Wiesbaden.

Klüver, H., & Bäck, H. (2019). Coalition Agreements, Issue Attention, and Cabinet Governance. *Comparative Political Studies, 52*(13-14), 1995–2031. https://doi.org/10.1177/0010414019830726

Knieps, F. (2009). Evidence Based Health Policy oder wissenschaftlich verbrämter Lobbyismus – Die Verwertung wissenschaftlicher Erkenntnisse in der Gesundheitspolitik. *Zeitschrift für Evidenz, Fortbildung und Qualität im Gesundheitswesen, 103*(5), 273–280. https://doi.org/10.1016/j.zefq.2009.05.003

Kube, H. (2004). Zehn Thesen für Demokratie und Reformfähigkeit in Deutschland. *Zeitschrift für Rechtspolitik, 37*(2), 52–55. Retrieved from http://www.jstor.org/stable/23428262

Kuhlmann, J., & van der Heijden, J. (2018). What Is Known about Punctuated Equilibrium Theory? And What Does That Tell Us about the Construction, Validation, and Replication of Knowledge in the Policy Sciences? *Review of Policy Research, 35*(2), 326–347. https://doi.org/10.1111/ropr.12283

Lazardeux, S. G. (2009). The French National Assembly's Oversight of the Executive: Changing Role, Partisanship and Intra-Majority Conflict. *West European Politics, 32*(2), 287–309. https://doi.org/10.1080/014 02380802670578

Lazardeux, S. G. (2015). Cohabitation and Policymaking Efficiency: An Empirical Test. In S. G. Lazardeux (Ed.), *Cohabitation and Conflicting Politics in French Policymaking* (pp. 88–111). Palgrave Macmillan UK.

Lehmbruch, G. (1977). Liberal Corporatism and Party Government. *Comparative Political Studies, 10*(1), 91–126. https://doi.org/10.1177/00104140 7701000105

Lehmbruch, G. (1998). *Parteienwettbewerb im Bundesstaat. Regelsysteme und Spannungslagen im Institutionengefüge der Bundesrepublik Deutschland.* Springer VS.

Leiber, S., Greß, S., & Manouguian, M.-S. (2010). Health Care System Change and the Cross-Border Transfer of Ideas: Influence of the Dutch Model on the 2007 German Health Reform. *Journal of Health Politics, Policy and Law, 35*(4), 539–568. https://doi.org/10.1215/03616878-2010-016

Leiser, S. (2015). The Diffusion of State Tax Incentives for Business. *Public Finance Review, 45*(3), 334–363. https://doi.org/10.1177/1091142 115611741

Lijphart, A. (2012). *Patterns of Democracy: Government Forms and Performance in Thirty-Six Countries* (2nd ed.). Yale Univ. Press.

Lijphart, A., & Crepaz, M. M. L. (1991). Corporatism and Consensus Democracy in Eighteen Countries: Conceptual and Empirical Linkages. *British Journal of Political Science, 21*(2), 235–246. https://doi.org/10.1017/S0007123400 006128

Löblová, O. (2016). Three Worlds of Health Technology Assessment: Explaining Patterns of Diffusion of HTA Agencies in Europe. *Health Economics, Policy and Law, 11*(3), 253–273. https://doi.org/10.1017/S1744133115000444

Lux, J. (2015). France in Limbo: On the Struggles Over Accumulation Strategies in Models of Capitalism – The Case of the Pacte de Responsabilité. *French Politics, 13*(1), 84–102. https://doi.org/10.1057/fp.2015.1

Maggetti, M., & Gilardi, F. (2016). Problems (and Solutions) in the Measurement of Policy Diffusion Mechanisms. *Journal of Public Policy, 36*(1), 87–107. https://doi.org/10.1017/S0143814X1400035X

Maillard, J. D., & Kübler, D. (2015). *Analyser Les Politiques Publiques.* Presses Universitaires de Grenoble.

Makse, T. (2020). Expertise and the Championing of Policy Innovations in State Legislatures. *Policy Studies Journal, n/a*(n/a). doi:https://doi.org/10.1111/psj.12380

Makse, T., & Volden, C. (2011). The Role of Policy Attributes in the Diffusion of Innovations. *The Journal of Politics, 73*(1), 108–124. https://doi.org/10.1017/S0022381610000903

Manow, P., & Burkhart, S. (2011). Legislative Self-Restraint Under Divided Government In Germany, 1976–2002. *Legislative Studies Quarterly, 32*(2), 167–191. https://doi.org/10.3162/036298007780907941

March, J. G., & Olsen, J. P. (2008). Elaborating the "New Institutionalism". In S. A. Binder, R. A. W. Rhodes, & B. A. Rockman (Eds.), *The Oxford Handbook of Political Institutions* (pp. 3–20). Oxford University Press.

Marmor, T. R., & Thomas, D. (1972). Doctors, Politics and Pay Disputes: 'Pressure Group Politics' Revisited. *British Journal of Political Science, 2*(4), 421–442. https://doi.org/10.1017/S0007123400008796

Marsh, D., & Sharman, J. C. (2009). Policy Diffusion and Policy Transfer. *Policy Studies, 30*(3), 269–288. https://doi.org/10.1080/01442870902863851

Martinsen, D. S., Schrama, R., & Mastenbroek, E. (2020). Experimenting European Healthcare Forward. Do Institutional Differences Condition Networked Governance? *Journal of European Public Policy, 1,* 1–22. https://doi.org/10.1080/13501763.2020.1804436

Marx, P., & Schumacher, G. (2013). Will to Power? Intra-party Conflict in Social Democratic Parties and the Choice for Neoliberal Policies in Germany, the Netherlands and Spain (1980–2010). *European Political Science Review, 5*(1), 151–173. https://doi.org/10.1017/S1755773912000070

Mazevet, M. E., Garyga, V., Pitts, N. B., & Pennington, M. W. (2018). The Highly Controversial Payment Reform of Dentists in France: Seeking a New Compromise After the 2017 Strike. *Health Policy, 122*(12), 1273–1277. https://doi.org/10.1016/j.healthpol.2018.10.001

McComas, K. A., Tuite, L. S., & Sherman, L. A. (2005). Conflicted Scientists: the "Shared Pool" Dilemma of Scientific Advisory Committees. *Public Understanding of Science, 14*(3), 285–303. https://doi.org/10.1177/0963662505052891

Mendy, A. F. (2015). Institutional Legacies, Employment and Professional Integration of Non-EU/EEA Doctors in France. *International Migration Institute (IMI) Working Paper, 188,* 1–24.

Mertens, A., Trampusch, C., Fastenrath, F., & Wangemann, R. (2019). The Political Economy of Local Government Financialization and the Role of Policy Diffusion. *Regulation & Governance, n/a*(n/a). doi:https://doi.org/10.1111/rego.12285

Michel, É. (2008). Verfassungreform in Frankreich: Eine neue Rolle für das Parlament? *Deutscher Bundestag - Wissenschaftliche Dienste, 27*(08), 1–4.

Mills, C. W. (2000). *The Power Elite.* Oxford University Press.

Mitchell, J. L. (2018). Does Policy Diffusion Need Space? Spatializing the Dynamics of Policy Diffusion. *Policy Studies Journal, 46*(2), 424–451. https://doi.org/10.1111/psj.12226

Molina, O., & Rhodes, M. (2002). CORPORATISM: The Past, Present, and Future of a Concept. *Annual Review of Political Science, 5*(1), 305–331. https://doi.org/10.1146/annurev.polisci.5.112701.184858

Morin, J.-F., & Gold, E. R. (2014). An Integrated Model of Legal Transplantation: The Diffusion of Intellectual Property Law in Developing Countries*. *International Studies Quarterly, 58*(4), 781–792. https://doi.org/10.1111/isqu.12176

Mosley, L., & Uno, S. (2007). Racing to the Bottom or Climbing to the Top? Economic Globalization and Collective Labor Rights. *Comparative Political Studies, 40*(8), 923–948. https://doi.org/10.1177/0010414006293442

Müller-Rommel, F. (1997). Federal Republic of Germany: A System of Chancellor Government. In J. Blondel & F. Müller-Rommel (Eds.), *Cabinets in Western Europe* (pp. 171–191). Palgrave Macmillan UK.

Navarro, J., Vaillant, N. G., & Wolff, F.-C. (2012). Measuring Parliamentary Effectiveness in the French National Assembly. The Contribution of Non-parametric Frontier Methods. *Revue française de science politique, 62*(4), 611–636. https://doi.org/10.3917/rfsp.624.0611

Nicholson-Crotty, S., & Carley, S. (2015). Effectiveness, Implementation, and Policy Diffusion: Or "Can We Make That Work for Us?". *State Politics & Policy Quarterly, 16*(1), 78–97. https://doi.org/10.1177/1532440015588764

O'Reilly, R. F. (2005). Veto Points, Veto Players, and International Trade Policy. *Comparative Political Studies, 38*(6), 652–675. https://doi.org/10.1177/0010414004274379

Obinger, H., Schmitt, C., & Starke, P. (2013). Policy Diffusion and Policy Transfer in Comparative Welfare State Research. *Social Policy & Administration, 47*(1), 111–129. https://doi.org/10.1111/spol.12003

Parsons, S. (1988). On the Logic of Corporatism. *Political Studies, 36*(3), 515–523. https://doi.org/10.1111/j.1467-9248.1988.tb00246.x

Pasquino, G. (2005). Duverger and the Study of Semi-Presidentialism. *French Politics, 3*(3), 310–322. https://doi.org/10.1057/palgrave.fp.8200081

Peters, B. G. (1996). Political Institutions, Old and New. In R. E. Goodin & H.-D. Klingemann (Eds.), *A New Handbook of Political Science* (pp. 180–193). Oxford University Press Inc.

Peterson, M. A. (2018). In the Shadow of Politics: The Pathways of Research Evidence to Health Policy Making. *Journal of Health Politics Policy and Law, 43*, 341–376.

Pierson, P. (1995). Fragmented Welfare States: Federal Institutions and the Development of Social Policy. *Governance, 8*(4), 449–478.

Price, D. K. (1943). The Parliamentary and Presidential Systems. *Public Administration Review, 3*(4), 317–334. https://doi.org/10.2307/972312

Propper, C. (2018). Competition in Health Care: Lessons From the English Experience. *Health Economics, Policy and Law, 13*(3-4), 492–508. https://doi.org/10.1017/S1744133117000494

Putnam, R. D. (1976). *The Comparative Study of Political Elites*. Prentice Hall.

Rhodes, R. A. W., 't Hart, P., & Noordegraaf, M. (2007). Being There. In R. A. W. Rhodes, P. 't Hart, & M. Noordegraaf (Eds.), *Observing Government Elites. Up Close and Personal* (pp. 1–17). Palgrave Macmillan.

Roberts, J. J., Lightbody, R., Low, R., & Elstub, S. (2020). Experts and Evidence in Deliberation: Scrutinising the Role of Witnesses and Evidence in Mini-publics, a Case Study. *Policy Sciences, 53*(1), 3–32. https://doi.org/10.1007/s11077-019-09367-x

Rouban, L. (2007). Public Management and Politics: Senior Bureaucrats in France. *Public Administration, 85*(2), 473–501. https://doi.org/10.1111/j.1467-9299.2007.00644.x

Saalfeld, T., Bahr, M., & Seifert, O. (2019). Contractual Arrangements, Formal Institutions and Personalised Crisis Management: Coalition Governance Under Chancellor Merkel (2013–2017). *German Politics, 28*(3), 371–391. https://doi.org/10.1080/09644008.2018.1512591

Saikawa, E. (2013). Policy Diffusion of Emission Standards. Is There a Race to the Top? *World Politics, 65*(1), 1–33. https://doi.org/10.1017/S00438871 12000238

Saltman, R. B. (1997). The Context for Health Reform in the United Kingdom, Sweden, Germany, and the United States. *Health Policy, 41*, S9–S26. https://doi.org/10.1016/S0168-8510(97)00050-X

Saretzki, T. (2019). Evidence-based Policy-making? The Meaning of Scientific Knowledge in Policy Processes. *Zeitschrift für Evidenz, Fortbildung und Qualität im Gesundheitswesen, 144*, 78–83. https://doi.org/10.1016/j.zefq.2019.05.008

Saurugger, S., & Terpan, F. (2016). Do Crises Lead to Policy Change?: The Multiple Streams Framework and the European Union's Economic Governance Instruments. *Policy Sciences, 49*(1), 35–53. https://doi.org/10.1007/s11077-015-9239-4

Schmidt, M. G. (2002). Political Performance and Types of Democracy: Findings from Comparative Studies. *European Journal of Political Research, 41*(1), 147–163.

Schmidt, M. G. (2008). Germany: The Grand Coalition State. In J. M. Colomer (Ed.), *Comparative European Politics*. Routledge.

Schmitter, P. C. (1974). Still the Century of Corporatism? *The Review of Politics, 36*(1), 85–131. https://doi.org/10.1017/S0034670500022178

Schreyögg, J., Tiemann, O., & Busse, R. (2006). Cost Accounting to Determine Prices: How Well Do Prices Reflect Costs in the German DRG-system? *Health Care Management Science, 9*(3), 269–279. https://doi.org/10.1007/s10729-006-9094-0

Schubert, K., & Bandelow, N. C. (Eds.). (2014). *Lehrbuch der Politikfeldanalyse* (3., aktualisierte und überarb. Aufl. ed.). München: De Gruyter Oldenbourg.

Schumacher, G., & van Kersbergen, K. (2014). Do Mainstream Parties Adapt to the Welfare Chauvinism of Populist Parties? *Party Politics, 22*(3), 300–312. https://doi.org/10.1177/1354068814549345

Searls, E. (1978). The Fragmented French Executive: Ministerial Cabinets in the Fifth Republic. *West European Politics, 1*(2), 161–176. https://doi.org/10.1080/01402387808424198

Seeleib-Kaiser, M. (2010). Socio-Economic Change, Party Competition and Intra-Party Conflict: The Family Policy of the Grand Coalition. *German Politics, 19*(3-4), 416–428. https://doi.org/10.1080/09644008.2010.515789

Seixas, C., & Costa, M. L. (2021). Paths to Power and Ministers' Durability: The Portuguese Case. *West European Politics, 44*(2), 403–425. https://doi.org/1 0.1080/01402382.2019.1687232

Shaw, R., & Eichbaum, C. (2020). Bubbling Up or Cascading Down? Public Servants, Political Advisers and Politicization. *Public Administration, 98*(4), 840–855. https://doi.org/10.1111/padm.12659

Shields, J. G. (2005). Political Representation in France: A Crisis of Democracy? *Parliamentary Affairs, 59*(1), 118–137. https://doi.org/10.1093/pa/gsj013

Shipan, C. R., & Volden, C. (2008). The Mechanisms of Policy Diffusion. *American Journal of Political Science, 52*(4), 840–857. https://doi. org/10.1111/j.1540-5907.2008.00346.x

Starke, P., & Tosun, J. (2019). Globalisierung und Diffusion. In H. Obinger & M. G. Schmidt (Eds.), *Handbuch Sozialpolitik* (pp. 181–201). Springer Fachmedien Wiesbaden.

Stecker, C. (2016). The Effects of Federalism Reform on the Legislative Process in Germany. *Regional & Federal Studies, 26*(5), 603–624. https://doi.org/1 0.1080/13597566.2016.1236334

Steiner, N. D., & Mader, M. (2017). Intra-Party Heterogeneity in Policy Preferences and its Effect on Issue Salience: Developing and Applying a Measure based on Elite Survey Data. *Party Politics*, 1354068817715553. doi:https://doi.org/10.1177/1354068817715553

Strang, D., & Meyer, J. W. (1993). Institutional Conditions for Diffusion. *Theory and Society, 22*(4), 487–511. https://doi.org/10.1007/BF00993595

Suleiman, E. N. (1974). *Politics, Power, and Bureaucracy in France. The Administrative Elite*. Princeton University Press.

Toens, K. (2008). Between Corporatism and Lobbyism. German Welfare Associations in Transition. *German Policy Studies, 4*(2), 101–130.

Trampusch, C. (2020). The Politics of Shifting Burdens: German Fiscal Welfare Corporatism. In R. Careja, P. Emmenegger, & N. Giger (Eds.), *The European Social Model under Pressure: Liber Amicorum in Honour of Klaus Armingeon* (pp. 159–176). Springer Fachmedien Wiesbaden.

Tranthimy, L. (2019). Déserts, Hôpitaux: La Santé s'est Invitée dans le Grand Débat, même Edouard Philippe le Reconnait. *Le Quotidien Du Medecin.*

Tsebelis, G. (1995). Decision Making in Political Systems: Veto Players in Presidentialism, Parliamentarism, Multicameralism and Multipartyism. *British Journal of Political Science, 25*(3), 289–325. https://doi.org/10.1017/ S0007123400007225

Tsebelis, G. (1999). Veto Players and Law Production in Parliamentary Democracies: An Empirical Analysis. *American Political Science Review, 93*(3), 591–608. https://doi.org/10.2307/2585576

Tsebelis, G. (2000). Veto Players and Institutional Analysis. *Governance, 13*(4), 441–474. https://doi.org/10.1111/0952-1895.00141

Tsebelis, G. (2002). *Veto Players: How Political Institutions Work.* Princeton University Press.

Tsebelis, G., & Chang, E. C. C. (2004). Veto Players and the Structure of Budgets in Advanced Industrialized Countries. *European Journal of Political Research, 43*(3), 449–476. https://doi.org/10.1111/j.1475-6765.2004.00161.x

Ulrich, V. (2012). Entwicklung der Gesundheitsökonomie in Deutschland. *Bundesgesundheitsblatt - Gesundheitsforschung - Gesundheitsschutz, 55*(5), 604–613. https://doi.org/10.1007/s00103-012-1478-3

Verspohl, I. (2012). *Health Care Reforms in Europe: Convergence towards a Market Model?* (1st ed.). Nomos Verlagsgesellschaft mbH & Co. KG.

Verzichelli, L. (2018). Executive Elites. In H. Best & J. Higley (Eds.), *The Palgrave Handbook of Political Elites.* Macmillan Publishers Ltd.

Volden, C. (2017). Policy Diffusion in Polarized Times: The Case of the Affordable Care Act. *Journal of Health Politics, Policy and Law, 42*(2), 363–375. https://doi.org/10.1215/03616878-3766762

von Beyme, K. (1983). Neo-Corporatism: A New Nut in an Old Shell? *International Political Science Review, 4*(2), 173–196. https://doi.org/10.1177/019251218300400204

von Winter, T. (2014). Dimensionen des Korporatismus. Strukturmuster der Verbändebeteiligung in der Gesundheitspolitik. In T. von Winter & J. von Blumenthal (Eds.), *Interessengruppen und Parlamente* (pp. 179–209). Springer Fachmedien Wiesbaden.

Weible, C. M., & Sabatier, P. A. (Eds.). (2017). *Theories of the Policy Process* (4th ed.). Westview Press.

Wenzelburger, G. (2011). Political Strategies and Fiscal Retrenchment: Evidence from Four Countries. *West European Politics, 34*(6), 1151–1184. https://doi.org/10.1080/01402382.2011.572385

Wenzelburger, G., & Zohlnhöfer, R. (2014). Institutionen und Public Policies. In K. Schubert & N. C. Bandelow (Eds.), *Lehrbuch der Politikfeldanalyse* (pp. 311–340). De Gruyter Oldenbourg.

Wenzelburger, G., & Zohlnhöfer, R. (Eds.). (2015). *Handbuch Policy-Forschung.* Springer Fachmedien Wiesbaden.

Weßels, B. (2007). Das bundesdeutsche Verbandssystem in vergleichender Perspektive. Politische Spannungslinien und politische Ökonomie. In T. von Winter & U. Willems (Eds.), *Interessenverbände in Deutschland* (pp. 84–118). VS Verlag für Sozialwissenschaften.

Willems, E. (2020). Politicized Policy Access: The Effect of Politicization on Interest Group Access to Advisory Councils. *Public Administration, 98*(4), 856–872. https://doi.org/10.1111/padm.12651

Wilsford, D. (1991). *Doctors and the State: the Politics of Health Care in France and the United States.* Duke University Press.

Wolkenstein, F., Senninger, R., & Bischof, D. (2019). Party Policy Diffusion in the European Multilevel Space: What It Is, How It Works, and Why It Matters. *Journal of Elections, Public Opinion and Parties, 1*, 19. https://doi.org/1 0.1080/17457289.2019.1666403

Zohlnhöfer, R. (2003). Partisan Politics, Party Competition and Veto Players: German Economic Policy in the Kohl Era. *Journal of Public Policy, 23*(2), 123–156. https://doi.org/10.1017/s0143814x03003064

Zohlnhöfer, R., Herweg, N., & Huß, C. (2016). Bringing Formal Political Institutions into the Multiple Streams Framework: An Analytical Proposal for Comparative Policy Analysis. *Journal of Comparative Policy Analysis: Research and Practice, 18*(3), 243–256. https://doi.org/10.1080/1387698 8.2015.1095428

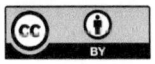

CHAPTER 4

Health Policy Institutions in France and Germany

Before being able to assess the impact of institutional on programmatic action, it is necessary to present an overview of the institutions found in French and German health care systems. This allows for performing a systematic analysis of how these play out in policy processes. The subsequent two chapters provide an overview of the institutions of French and German health policy, with a particular focus on the institutions for which the previous chapter has formulated hypotheses.

4.1 Institutions of French Health Policy: Centralization, Education, and Advice

In 2000, the French health care system was recognized by the World Health Organization as the best in the world in terms of quality and provision (Schütte et al., 2018, p. 4). Recent typologies refer to the French health care system as an "Etatist Social Health Insurance type" (Böhm et al., 2013, p. 264), indicating a "technocratic civil service elite" (Freeman, 1998, p. 398) that supports a centralized system of decision-making. Yet, typologies of health care systems tend to represent ideal types that are useful as starting points but do not take into account the fullness of institutional complexity (Burau & Blank, 2006, p. 74). Categorizing the French (or German) health care system into highly simplified structures falls short of achieving a deep understanding of the institutions and processes that organize health care, which is the goal of this chapter.

© The Author(s) 2022   113
J. Hornung, *The Institutions of Programmatic Action*,
International Series on Public Policy,
https://doi.org/10.1007/978-3-031-05774-8_4

Despite the frequent label of centralization and hierarchical governance, the French health care system was originally rooted in an organization based on municipal structures without noteworthy state intervention, except for epidemic control and municipal governance failures. The establishment of sickness funds in 1928 and 1930 and a fixed social security system in 1945 presented the first steps toward increased autonomization of health care units. These developments culminated in regulations issued by decree in 1967, through the Plan Juppé 1996, to the 2016 Health System Modernization Act, which placed state actors even more at the center of responsibility for health care (Tabuteau, 2010).

The French health care system is based on a contribution-financed health insurance, co-financed by employers and employees, and provides universal health coverage for all citizens through three main insurance schemes, with the general SHI scheme (Caisse Nationale d'Assurance Maladie des Travailleurs Salariés; CNAMTS) covering more than 90% of the French population. The representative for all sickness funds is the National Union of Health Insurance Funds (Union Nationale des Caisses d'Assurance Maladie; UNCAM) (Chevreul et al., 2015, p. 29). The reimbursement principle and free choice of physician apply. However, since 2004, there has been requirement to consult a primary care physician before consulting a specialist. Failure to do so can result in a drop in reimbursement by the health insurance companies from 70% to 40% (Tinapp & Hesselbarth, 2019, p. 33).

The most important institution in the process of health policy-making is the health ministry and—for formal legislation—the parliament. Within the administrative structure of the ministry, some units appear to be particularly relevant for policy formulation. These are the Directorate of Social Security (Direction de la Sécurité Sociale; DSS), the General Directorate of Health Care Supplies (Direction Générale de l'Offre de Soins; DGOS), and the General Directorate of Health (Direction Générale de Santé, DGS). Finally, the General Inspectorate for Social Affairs (Inspection Générale des Affaires Sociales; IGAS) is a central body. Also located within the ministry's internal structures, it is regularly tasked with investigating and evaluating policies and administrative structures and is an important source of expert advice to both the health ministry and the public, as its reports are publicly available (IGAS, 2020).

In addition to the health ministry and—to a lesser extent—the parliament, the health policy process is dominated by a variety of advisory bodies and the involvement of expert advice. These include the High Council for the Future of Health Insurance (Haut Conseil pour l'Avenir de l'Assurance Maladie; HCAAM), the High Council for Public Health (Haut Conseil de la Santé Publique; HCSP) (former High Committee for Public Health (Haut Comité de la Santé Publique, HCSP)), and the National Health Conference (Conférence Nationale de Santé; CNS), which regularly issue reports on the health care system on the basis of which key decisions are made, such as the annual social security budget (Chevreul et al., 2015, pp. 23-25). In particular, the HCAAM and the CNS provide an interface between the ministry and the UNCAM. While formally attached to the ministry, they are composed of a range of subsystem actors, including health care providers and payers, scientific institutes, unions, and other public and private health care actors. Moreover, they are essentially involved in the development of ideas and the translation of those ideas into concrete policy proposals, thereby influencing the policy-making process through the health ministry (CNS, 2020; HCAAM, 2020).

It is striking that, apart from the central role of the UNCAM, other health care actors are almost excluded from decision-making processes at the federal level (with exceptions at the regional level). Nevertheless, there is a historically important role of physicians' associations, which at times have been able to block major reforms (Hassenteufel, 1996). French physicians—comparable to those in other countries—highly value their freedom and professional autonomy, making them a natural enemy of constrained competencies and regulation by the state. Despite this potential veto position, the fragmentation of physicians' associations has enabled governments to overcome these blockades (Immergut, 1992). Although physicians were able to take back regulations adopted in the mid-1990s, for example on reimbursement for exceeding cost caps, the fragmentation of associations remains not only an impeding factor but also a driving factor for major health reforms (Brunn & Hassenteufel, 2018).

The UNCAM has considerable power in setting drug reimbursement prices and negotiating contracts with providers, particularly physicians' associations. Nevertheless, this power is formal rather than de facto, as the ministry has the authority to decide on the admission of drugs and as the reimbursement rate is also subject to a decree by the minister (Grandfils, 2008, p. 18). Although these decisions are based on the advice of the National Health Authority (Haute Autorité de Santé; HAS) (Goujard, 2018, p. 32) and are guided by the evaluation criteria of evidence-based medicine, the health ministry intervenes regularly (Ansaloni et al., 2018). Thus, following the French centralist state model, decision-making is highly hierarchical. The main structures of decision-making in French health policy are shown in a simplified form in Fig. 4.1.

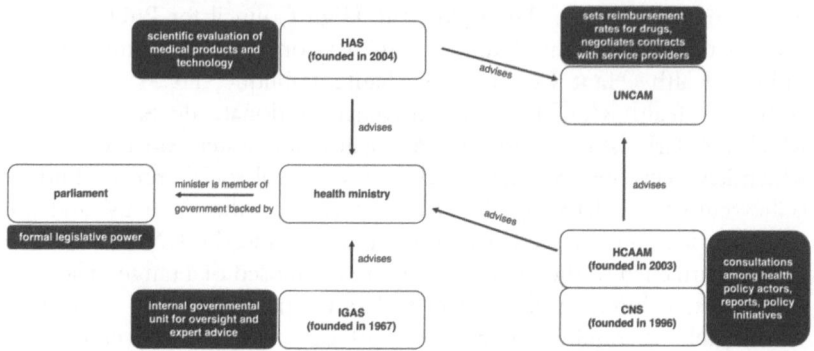

Fig. 4.1 Institutions with direct access to decision-making processes in French health policy. Source: Simplified and slightly modified overview on the basis of Chevreul et al. (2015, p. 21)

In summary, the French health care system, like the political system, is characterized by hierarchical structures of policy-making with a remarkably high degree of institutionalized and regular exchange among actors directly involved in health care and combined with a high level of expertise.

4.2   Institutions of German Health Policy: Self-Governance and Corporatism

Although the French and German health care systems are considered prototypes of Bismarckian, that is, contribution-based health insurance systems with compulsory health insurance and universal coverage, the two Bismarckian systems differ considerably. This is not only because the German system is a divided insurance system with the co-existence of statutory and private health insurance. In particular, the history and path dependencies of the two systems differ with regard to the different involvement and organization of medical interests and health insurance actors, the much greater relevance of the employee-employer conflict in France compared to Germany, and the centralized versus decentralized modes of decision-making (Steffen, 2010, pp. 145-148). Comparing the institutional setting of German health policy with the previously elaborated French health care system, these institutional differences become even more apparent. The relevant German health sector institutions are shown in Fig. 4.2.

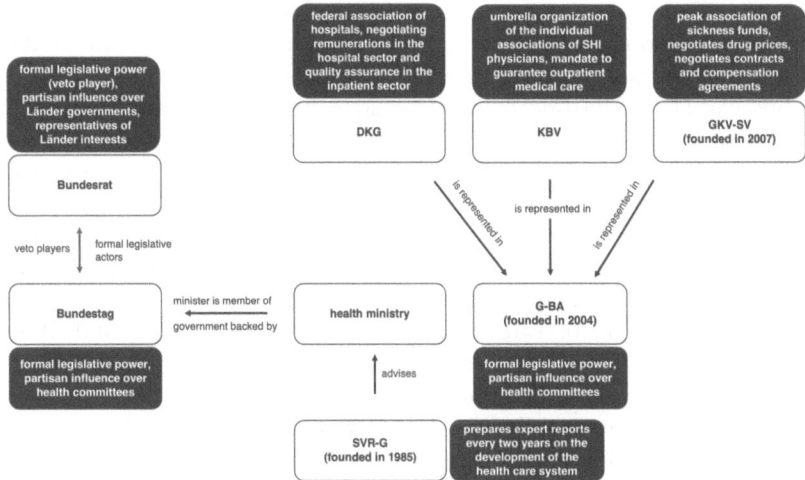

Fig. 4.2 Institutions with direct access to decision-making processes in German health policy. Source: Simplified and modified overview on the basis of Busse and Blümel (2014, p. 18)

Although the health ministry and the parliament, with their formal legislative power, play as central a role in Germany as they do in France, and although there are several expert bodies that inform health policy decisions, the institutional conditions under which health policy is made are different. First, because of the German political system, the Federal Council has veto power over health policy decisions that affect subnational competences. These competences lie primarily in the organization of inpatient care, with a central role of hospital planning committees. Even when there are no formal competences in certain areas, the subnational states exert an influence on health policy. Their own ministries and the coordination of health ministries at the subnational level can take the form of think tanks and preparatory as well as experimental laboratories for certain policies before they are placed on the party-political or federal ministerial agenda (Bandelow et al., 2012). Some sickness funds are also subject to subnational rather than federal supervision, which allows subnational states to set different rules than at the federal level (Orlowski, 2008).

In addition to the stronger role of the subnational level, the corporatist structures of the German health care system also differ from the French health care system. The German health care system is characterized by a specific role of self-governance, its multilateral negotiations, and resulting binding decisions among actors of the self-governance. The status of the associations of sickness funds types and the associations of medical professions has grown historically and the state has deliberately given them the remit to guarantee the provision of health care services (Sicherstellungsauftrag), which in the corporatist tradition trades increased responsibility for the need for negotiating consensus. As a consequence, a substantial role for physicians' associations is foreseen. Since the introduction of selective contracts, the role of sickness funds and physicians' associations has been further strengthened by granting them the right to negotiate local health care contracts (Jacobs, 2020). The SHI Peak Association (GKV-Spitzenverband, GKV-SV) has a special role in negotiating prices for health care provision and pharmaceuticals (Schnorpfeil & Gassner, 2020) with the Federal Association of Sickness Fund Physicians (Kassenärztliche Bundesvereinigung; KBV) at the federal level.

The most important decision-making body of self-governance is the Federal Joint Committee (Gemeinsamer Bundesausschuss, G-BA). Excluding its impartial members, the providers (hospitals and physicians, German Hospital Association (Deutsche Krankenhausgesellschaft, DKG) and KBV) and payers (health insurance funds) of health care each have five votes and, by definition, oppose each other. The G-BA is responsible for selecting the range of services to be reimbursed by the SHI system, evaluating methods according to the criteria of evidence-based medicine, and promoting innovative forms of care through the Innovation Fund (G-BA, 2020). While the individual benches sometimes represent very strong interests that are reflected in debates about problems and adequate solutions for German health policy, the institution of the G-BA itself is a decision-making and implementation body that rarely promotes certain reform proposals on its own initiative and as a unit—not least because the G-BA cannot represent uniformly determined positions.

The most prominent advisory body to German health policy with regard to the systematic involvement of scientific advice is the Council of Experts on the Assessment of Developments in the Health Care System (Sachverständigenrat zur Begutachtung der Entwicklung im Gesundheitswesen, SVR-G). Formally located at the health ministry, it produces expert reports that analyze challenges and propose solutions for important developments in the health care system. Its members often comprise health economists and physicians. Since they are based in the health ministry, they have a direct link to the decision-making structures.

References

Ansaloni, M., Pariente, A., & Smith, A. (2018). Power Shifts in the Regulation of Medicines: an Inter-field Analysis of a French Agency. *Critical Policy Studies, 12*(3), 314–334. https://doi.org/10.1080/19460171.2017.1314220

Bandelow, N. C., Eckert, F., & Rüsenberg, R. (2012). Wie funktioniert Gesundheitspolitik? In B. Klein & M. Weller (Eds.), *Masterplan Gesundheitswesen 2020* (pp. 37–62). Nomos.

Böhm, K., Schmid, A., Götze, R., Landwehr, C., & Rothgang, H. (2013). Five Types of OECD Healthcare Systems: Empirical Results of a Deductive Classification. *Health Policy, 113*(3), 258–269. https://doi.org/10.1016/j.healthpol.2013.09.003

Brunn, M., & Hassenteufel, P. (2018). Frankreich: Gesundheitspolitik weiter "en marche?". *Gesundheits- und Sozialpolitik, 72*(3), 7–12.

Burau, V., & Blank, R. H. (2006). Comparing Health Policy: An Assessment of Typologies of Health Systems. *Journal of Comparative Policy Analysis: Research and Practice, 8*(1), 63–76. https://doi.org/10.1080/13876980500513558

Busse, R., & Blümel, M. (2014). *Germany: Health System Review*. WHO Regional Off. for Europe.

Chevreul, K., Berg Brigham, K., Durand-Zaleski, I., & Hernández-Quevedo, C. (2015). *France: Health System Review*. WHO Regional Off. for Europe.

CNS, L. C. N. d. S. (2020). Fiche de Présentation. *https://solidarites-sante.gouv. fr/IMG/pdf/fiche_presentation_cns_090320.pdf (last retrieved from 3 July 2020)*.

Freeman, R. (1998). Competition in Context: the Politics of Health Care Reform in Europe. *International Journal for Quality in Health Care, 10*(5), 395–401. https://doi.org/10.1093/intqhc/10.5.395

G-BA, G. B. (2020). Der Gemeinsame Bundesausschuss. *https://www.g-ba.de/ ueber-den-gba/wer-wir-sind/ (last retrieved from 21 April 2020)*.

Goujard, A. (2018). France: Improving the Efficiency of the Health-Care System. *OECD Economics Department Working Papers, 1455*, 2-50. doi:https://doi.org/10.1787/09e92b30-en

Grandfils, N. (2008). Drug Price Setting and Regulation in France. *Working Paper / Institut de recherche et documentation en économie de la santé DT n° 16*(https://core.ac.uk/download/pdf/6549409.pdf (last retrieved from 3 July 2020)).

Hassenteufel, P. (1996). The Medical Profession and Health Insurance Policies: A Franco-German Comparison. *Journal of European Public Policy, 3*(3), 461–480. https://doi.org/10.1080/13501769608407044

HCAAM, H. C. p. l. A. d. l. A. M. (2020). Sommaire. *https://www.securite-sociale. fr/hcaam (last retrieved from 3 July 2020)*.

IGAS, I. G. d. A. S. (2020). IGAS in brief. *http://www.igas.gouv.fr/spip. php?article490 (last retrieved from 3 July 2020)*.

Immergut, E. M. (1992). The Rules of the Game: The Logic of Health Policy-making in France, Switzerland, and Sweden. In F. Longstreth, K. Thelen, &

S. Steinmo (Eds.), *Structuring Politics: Historical Institutionalism in Comparative Analysis* (pp. 57–89). Cambridge University Press.

Jacobs, K. (2020). Vertragswettbewerb: Neustart geboten. *G&S Gesundheits- und Sozialpolitik, 74*(1), 24–28. https://doi.org/10.5771/1611-5821-2020-1-24

Orlowski, U. (2008). Gesundheitsfonds und Dachverband – wo steht die Krankenversicherung in fünf Jahren? In W. Voit (Ed.), *Gesundheitsreform 2007 - Rechtliche Bewertung und Handlungsoptionen: 10. Symposium von Wissenschaft und Praxis* (1 ed., pp. 66-72). Baden-Baden: Nomos Verlagsgesellschaft mbH & Co. KG.

Schnorpfeil, W., & Gassner, W. (2020). Preisverhandlungen in der GKV. In R. Tunder (Ed.), *Market Access Management für Pharma- und Medizinprodukte: Instrumente, Verfahren und Erfolgsfaktoren* (pp. 339–360). Springer Fachmedien Wiesbaden.

Schütte, S., Acevedo, P. N. M., & Flahault, A. (2018). Health Systems Around the World - A Comparison of Existing Health System Rankings. *Journal of Global Health, 8*(1), 010407–010407. https://doi.org/10.7189/jogh.08.010407

Steffen, M. (2010). Social Health Insurance Systems: What Makes the Difference? The Bismarckian Case in France and Germany. *Journal of Comparative Policy Analysis: Research and Practice, 12*(1-2), 141–161. https://doi.org/10.1080/13876980903076252

Tabuteau, D. (2010). Loi "Hôpital, Patients, Santé et Territoires" (HPST): des Interrogations Pour Demain! *Santé Publique, 22*(1), 78–90. https://doi.org/10.3917/spub.101.0078

Tinapp, C., & Hesselbarth, J. (2019). *Digitale Gesundheitswirtschaft - Schwerpunkt altersgerechte und pflegeunterstützende Technik*. Retrieved from Paris.

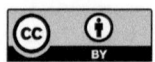

CHAPTER 5

Programmatic Action in French Health Policy

The analysis of the institutions that enabled French and German programmatic action takes as its starting point existing research on programmatic groups in health policy identified by existing studies. In the French case, there is an extensive body of research on the French welfare state elite, which implemented substantial health care reforms between 1990 and 2010 at minimum (Genieys & Hassenteufel, 2001; Hassenteufel et al., 2010). The following steps thus proceed through the formal research protocol for identifying potential programmatic groups in a policy area with the goal of laying the groundwork for identifying the programmatic actors to be interviewed in light of the central research question about the institutions of programmatic action. In doing so, the research steps take into account the identification of programmatic action in France and Germany in existing research.

5.1 POLICY PROGRAM IN FRENCH HEALTH POLICY

Looking at the laws that were passed and substantially reformed the health care system (Table 5.1), what can be observed as third-order policy change, and thus a major realignment, is the increasing use of a narrative that sees rising health care costs as the main problem and a centralization of competences with a stronger role of the state as the solution to this problem. In the early 1990s, some measures were taken in this direction,

© The Author(s) 2022
J. Hornung, *The Institutions of Programmatic Action*,
International Series on Public Policy,
https://doi.org/10.1007/978-3-031-05774-8_5

Table 5.1   Substantial health care reforms in France 1990–2010

Designation of reforms	Main reform content
LOI no 90-88 du 23 janvier 1990 portant diverses dispositions relatives à la sécurité sociale et à la santé (1)	Enables local and regional authorities to grant financial aid to provide incentives for the installation or maintenance of health care professionals in areas where health care provision is shortened
LOI no 91-739 du 31 Juillet 1991 portant diverses mesures d'ordre social (1)	Foresees an annual agreement between the ministry, the CNAMTS and at least one other health insurance fund and a representative trade union as representative for private hospitals to set a total annual amount of hospitalization costs
LOI no 91-748 du 31 Juillet 1991 portant réforme hospitalière (1)	Contains several measures to reorganize hospital structures, particularly by introducing a regional health organization scheme, planning the health care services both with regard to patient needs and cost containment, by relying on scientific advices and statistics, reduces hospital beds through restrictive planning to address rising hospital expenditures, strengthens the role of inter-hospital cooperation and unions and the board of directors of hospitals
LOI no 95-1348 du 30 décembre 1995 autorisant le Gouvernement, par application de l'article 38 de la Constitution, à réformer la protection sociale (1)	Presents the preparatory law to authorize the government to substantially reform the social security system, particularly with regard to the distribution of responsibilities and relations between bodies, professions, and insured, the financing structures and financial equilibrium with the aim of cost control, the establishment of new decision-making bodies, the rationalization of social security institutions
LOI no 95-452 du 28 mai 1996 portant diverses mesures d'ordre sanitaire, social et statutaire (1)	Strengthens IGAS (inspection générale des affaires sociales); responsible for monitoring and evaluating the implementation of public policies in the areas of social security and social welfare, health and social protection, labor, employment, and vocational training
LOI organique no 96-646 du 22 juillet 1996 relative aux lois de financement de la sécurité sociale (1)	Stipulates that the parliament is to adopt annually a law on the financing of social security, which includes orientations of health and social security policy and a set financial balance and budget for expenses of the national sickness funds. In that, it presents a preliminary balance of revenues and expenses of the compulsory schemes and sets for all of the national health insurance expenditures target (ONDAM)
LOI no 98-535 du 1er Juillet 1996 relative au renforcement de la veille sanitaire et du contrôle de la sécurité sanitaire des produits destines à l'homme	Specifies the scope and tasks of the French Agency of Health Security of Medical Products, replacing the Agency of Medicaments

(*continued*)

Table 5.1 (continued)

Designation of reforms	Main reform content
LOI no 2002-2 du 2 janvier 2002 rènovant l'action sociale et medico-sociale	Sets an expenditures target for the financing of benefits provided by public and private social and medico-social establishments and services which are the responsibility of social security bodies. This is annually determined by the responsible ministers for social security, social action, the economy and the budget, in accordance with the national health insurance expenditure target voted by parliament
LOI no 2002-322 du 6 mars 2002 portant renovation des rapports conventionnels entre les professions de santé liberals et les organismes d'assurance maladie	Specifies conditions for individual contracts between the health care providers and sickness funds; for the case of non-agreements, it grants the CNAMTS decisive rights for monitoring expenditures targets
LOI no 2004-810 du 13 aûot 2004 relative à l'assurance maladie	Establishes the Haute Autorité de Santé and specifies its constitution and scope of action; a health insurance expenditures alert committee is constituted and the scope of action is defined; a Hospitalization Council is hereby created, attached to the Ministers responsible for Health and Social Security. For the National Fund, a board and managing director are installed and their composition and scope of action are determined. Installs the Union nationale des caisses d'assurance maladie (National Union of Sickness Insurance Funds
LOI organique no 2005-881 du 2 août 2005 relative aux lois de financement de la sécurité sociale	Specifies further competences for the preparation of annual laws of the financing of the social security
Loi no 2006-337 du 15 avril 2006 ratifiant l'ordonannace no 2007-613 du 26 avril 2007 portant diverses dispositions d'adaption au droit communautaire dans le domaine du mèdicament	Increases control over medical products with respect to sanction in the event of failing to submit pharmaco-epidemiological studies thus strengthening the role of the French Agency of Health Security of Medical Products, replacing the Agency of Medicaments

(*continued*)

Table 5.1 (continued)

Designation of reforms	Main reform content
LOI no 2009-879 du 21 juillet 2009 portant rèforme de l'hôpital et relative aux patients, à la santé et aux teritoires	Creates regional health agencies, which organize access to primary care and ongoing care for the sick, replacing the Regional Health Agencies replace the Regional Hospitalization Agencies (ARH) created in 1996, which had the status of a public interest group. The ARss are also to replace other institutions from which they take over all or part of their remit, in particular the decentralized services of the Ministry of Health, namely the Regional Directorates of Health and Social Affairs (Directions regionals des Affaires sanitaires et sociales, DRASS) and the Departmental Directorates of Health and Social Affairs (Direction départementales des Affaires sanitaire et sociales (DDASS) and to replace certain social security bodies such as the Regional Unions of Health Insurance Funds and the Regional Health Insurance Funds (Union règionales des caisses d'assurance maladie et les Caisses regionals d'assurance malady, CRAM) More weight is given to the doctors and director in the governance of the hospital and the supervisory board

Source: République Française (2020)

based on negotiations between the social partners to achieve a reduction in health care spending.

However, these measures largely failed until the adoption of the so-called Plan Juppé, which is a reform that fundamentally restructured the health care system by introducing a universal health insurance system and giving parliament the annual task of setting an expenditure target for the national sickness funds (Bouget, 1998, p. 162; Lancry & Sandier, 1999). The so-called financing laws of the social security (Projet de loi de finance-ment de la Sécurité sociale, or PLFSS) are prepared each year by the DSS; this strengthens the role of the directorate and the state in social security financial decisions. In particular, since the preparation of this law and the DSS is under the double supervision of the health ministry and the finance ministry, this can be considered a key instrument for cost containment (Genieys & Hassenteufel, 2015, pp. 288-289). Other instruments of the Plan Juppé include the establishment of an annual national health conference attended by representatives of sectoral actors to prepare the annual finance law, and an administrative reform of the way the director of France's largest sickness fund, the CNAMTS, is appointed. This again increased state authority and oversight of sectoral actors. Other specific cost-control measures included the expansion of the social security income base subject to include capital income and the introduction of the "remboursement de la dette sociale"—a 0.5% tax on taxable income explicitly and exclusively intended to finance the deficit (Ruellan, 2015), as well as the creation of the CADES (Caisse d'Amortissement de la Dette Sociale; Social Debt Amortisation Fund) (Ract-Madoux & Gauthey, 2018).

The Plan Juppé met with strong opposition from the physicians' associations during its preparatory phase, especially because of the envisaged changes to a general practitioner-centered model of health care and an associated reform of physicians' remuneration (from a free basis to a contractual basis) and fixed budgets. In the course of their protests, the physicians' associations accused these measures of undermining the principle of "médecine libérale" and thus weakening the role of the physicians as self-employed entrepreneurs in a free economy.

Continuing the reforms that appealed to cost containment, the Douste-Blazy reform employed computerized patient records and a 1€ contact fee for a doctor's visit, along with charging for specialist treatment without prior consultation with a general practitioner, to control doctor visits and thus reduce costs. The reform also promoted the use of generic drugs, which are less expensive (Bosch, 2004), and created the National Union of Health Insurance Funds (Union Nationale des Caisses d'Assurance Maladie; UNCAM) as the representative body of the three major sickness funds. The director of UNCAM negotiates with the unions of physicians and other health professionals and signs medical agreements to meet health insurance spending targets set by parliament—a task previously assigned to the board of directors of the CNAMTS, whose director is now automatically also the director of UNCAM (Hassenteufel & Palier, 2005, p. 17). Both reforms also shifted decisive power from the social partners to the state, with centralization occurring through the merger of associations and the state's authority to appoint the directors of associations and thus shape positions of power (Hassenteufel & Palier, 2016, p. 68). These mergers and centralization of processes are often referred to as the solution to the challenge of a fragmented and diffuse nature of interest representation that was previously prevalent in the French health care sector. As a result of these preexisting structures, some policies lacked legitimacy among sectoral actors because they were negotiated and endorsed only by some interest unions but not by others, such as the reorganization of primary care through a "reference practitioner", a French model of general practitioner-centered health care.

These centralization ideas intellectually can be traced back to a commission chaired by Raymond Soubie, whose report strongly influenced not only the Plan Juppé but also the creation of regional hospital agencies (Agences Régionales de l'Hospitalisation; ARH) and their later successors, the regional health agencies (Agences Régionales de Santé, ARS), created in the course of the later 2009 HPST (Pierru & Rolland, 2016, p. 83). The latter was aimed at reorganizing regional care, particularly hospitals, and has been in preparation since Nicolas Sarkozy took office in 2007. The HPST reform was structurally designed to strengthen the state, primarily by tying hospital directors to the newly established regional health agencies (ARS). These act as an extension of the state and are equipped with the necessary competences to coordinate the regional health services and control related expenses (Grimaldi, 2015; Lopez, 2010, p. 567).

Researching a little deeper into the origins of these health care reforms, it becomes apparent that the reform ideas can be traced back to several working commissions within which these conceptions were worked out and to which the actors driving the reform process belonged. The first is the aforementioned planning commission chaired by Raymond Soubie, which was charged with conducting a prospective reflection on the future of the French health care system, resulting in a report called "Santé 2010" (Soubie et al., 1993). The work was done primarily through working groups led by Anne-Marie Brocas, Robert Rochefort, Christian Rollet/ Lise Rochaix, and Aïssa Khélifa (Bras & Tabuteau, 2009, p. 80). In essence, the commission's report put forward concrete proposals on cost containment, specifically on parliamentary control and the setting of an annual budget target. Related to this, the report also called for a fundamental restructuring of the health care system, in particular with regard to a centralization of the state's competences and a national administration defining the main lines of health policy and relies on a public institution (Bras & Tabuteau, 2009, p. 85). At the same time, a regionalization of health care and a centralization of decision-making and service provision through the merging of sickness funds and state services, and thus the creation of regional health service agencies, which then negotiate with the providers on prices, quantities, and quality of health care, is proposed (Bezat, 1993).

Cost containment measures had already been advocated by the same Raymond Soubie when he delivered the "Livre blanc sur le système de santé et d'assurance maladie" (White Paper on the Health and Health Insurance System) to then prime minister Balladur in December 1994

(Soubie et al., 1995). By this time, there were already several commissions, all of which had the task of evaluating the future of French policy sectors. Chief among these was a "Commission for the Evaluation of the Social, Economic and Financial Situation of France", which included bureaucrats and scientific advisors from a variety of disciplines (given the broad range of topics) and which included—in addition to Raymond Soubie—Jean Raynaud, Jacques Barel, Jean-Claude Casanova, Marguerite Gentzbittel, Lucien Israël, Pierre Laurent, Raymond Lévy, Jean Pinchon, Jean-Philippe Ricalens, Simon Rozes, Dominique Schnapper, and Guy Vidal (Treize membres., 1993) and a commission chaired by Alain Minc on "France in the year 2000" (members included Claude Bebear, Jean-Louis Beffa, Michel Bon, Isabelle Bouillot, Luc Ferry, Jean-Paul Fitoussi, Jean-Baptiste de Foucauld, Pierre Guillen, Rene Lenoir, Rene Remond, Pierre Rosanvallon, Raymond Soubie, and Alain Touraine) which proposed that the social partners also be involved in a major reform effort (Seux, 1994). The reports of Raymond Soubie and Alain Minc, as well as that of Philippe Lazar on ambulatory care in the regions, and the ideas of François-Xavier Stasse influenced the reform proposal pushed by Alain Juppé to regionalize health care while centralizing decision-making (Nouchi, 1995).

The HPST continued the ideational line of centralizing decision-making power by empowering hospital directors, as opposed to hospital boards of directors, to meet financial targets (Simonet, 2017, p. 3). One of the main components of the 2009 HPST reform under then health minister Roselyne Bachelot-Narquine was the creation of ARS. The report issued by the rapporteur Philippe Ritter in January 2008, entitled "Rapport sur la creation des agencies régionales de santé" (Report on the creation of regional health agencies), that announces this reform step explicitly refers to the origins of this policy idea. I quote the report (Ritter, 2008, p. 1) (translated):

- "the Minister has instructed [Philippe Ritter] to set up a mission to prepare for their creation, relying primarily on broad consultation with all the players concerned";
- "the result of this consultation, carried out with elected representatives, officials of the ministries concerned and of the health insurance, as well as with representatives of health professionals and users, but also of numerous reports and written contributions, this report presents a summary of the mission's work";

- "its content and recommendations have been the subject of regular discussions in particular with a working group made up of representatives of UNCAM and each of the administrative departments concerned, and with the steering committee for the reform, chaired by the minister, bringing together, in addition to the ministry, parliamentarians, representatives of the ministries of the interior, labour and the budget, and representatives of each of the health insurance schemes".

Therefore, one can conclude from this document that the policy idea at the core of the HPST reform was in fact the result of long-term preparation around a regularly meeting group of actors from various institutions that belonged directly to the state apparatus. But not only does the trajectory of this reform become clearer; the connection of the HPST reform with previous reform steps, in particular the Plan Juppé, is explicitly outlined in the introductory chapter. "The 1996 reform creating the ARH was a first step, which must now be completed and surpassed. The creation of ARS based on orderly cooperation between the State and the Health Insurance is one of the most important institutional reforms of recent decades" (Ritter, 2008, p. 2).

In addition and related to the creation of the ARS, the HPST included several other measures to facilitate collaboration among health institutions, particularly at the regional level (IRDES, 2018): For example, one or more public health establishments could join together to form territorial hospital communities (communautés hospitalières territoriales, CHT) and, through delegation or transfer of competences and telemedicine, implement a common strategy and jointly manage certain functions and activities. Such an agreement is subject to approval by the directors of the establishments, after consultation with their supervisory boards, and ultimately by the director general of the ARS. Another possibility for collaboration arose through so-called health cooperation and resource groups (groupements de coopération sanitaire de moyens, GCSM), which could be composed of public and private health establishments, medico-social establishments, health centers, and independent medical professionals working individually or in companies. The formation of such groups would, in turn, allow for the joint organization or management of administrative, logistical, technical, medico-technical, teaching, or research activities and would require approval by the director general of the

ARS. Finally, private health institutions are now less restricted in participating in public service provision, as this no longer depends on a special status. Under the label of private health establishments of collective interest (établissements de santé privés d'intérêt collectif (ESPIC)), private health institutions can register with the respective ARS either as cancer centers or as private health establishments managed by non-profit organizations (IRDES, 2018, pp. 8-12). In terms of cost containment, this inter-establishment collaboration between public and public, as well as private, facilities allow for more efficient use of resources and more responsive health care planning to regional needs. Overall, health care provision is organized more regionally than before, but it should not be confused with a decentralization of competences, as the ARS bundles various competences in a single institution that serves as an intermediary body to implement national guidelines and thus has only "relative autonomy" (Evin, 2019, p. 109). Nevertheless, policy ideas on the regionalization of health care can be traced back to the "Santé 2010" policy program.

Although many scholars of French health policy see the three reforms described above (Plan Juppé, Réforme Douste-Blazy, HPST) as the fundamental reforms in health care during the period under study, following a coherent vision for the policy sector (Hassenteufel, 2012; Palier, 2008, pp. 96-112; Ruellan, 2015), not all reforms in health policy can be attributed to the policy ideas and fit the substantive vision of the identified policy program. Some reforms did not explicitly pursue the goal of cost containment, but rather were the response to emerging problems, such as increased regulations following a contaminated blood scandal reveal.

In addition, the process of reducing the laws found under the keyword "santé" has removed from consideration some reforms that were related to other policy areas or specific areas of the policy sector, such as professional training and public health and prevention. However, these reforms may well belong to another policy program, possibly a cross-sectoral program aimed at combining environmental protection and public health, for example. In particular, some of the reforms between 1990 and 2010 also modified the code of public health (santé publique), for example, the "LOI n° 2004-806 du 9 août 2004 relative à la politique de santé publique (1)". Public health and prevention policies were also put on the agenda in the wake of the COVID-19 pandemic, which reached France in January 2020 and spread across Europe in March through June 2020 (Capano et al., 2020; Schrappe et al., 2020; Weible et al., 2020), although this already concerns the second period of analysis after 2010. Additionally, there are some reforms explicitly related to family and care policies and criminal justice policies, each of which could be indications of an underlying programmatic group.

Without neglecting the existence of other programmatic groups behind these thematic foci, further empirical analysis will focus on the structural reforms of the health insurance system in France, that is, the modification of the code of social security (code de la sécurité sociale), the substantial reorganization of the health care system, whose modifications were aimed at cost containment. This narrative description of the problem (inefficiency, rising costs) and the corresponding solution (setting annual targets for expenses, centralizing responsibility for meeting these targets, narrowing leeway for negotiating contracts between the social partners), which can be found in the reports and legal documents analyzed earlier, will also be kept in mind for the upcoming discourse analysis in search of the actors surrounding this narrative.

5.2   Programmatic Actors in French Health Policy

Tracing policy reforms back to ideational and personal roots allowed for an initial identification of substantial foci of policy reforms toward a potential policy program and the individuals who were mainly active in these ideational processes. This second step serves even more to explore the policy program as it appears not only in formal documents but also in public discourse. Therefore, in this subchapter, such discourse analysis will be conducted in relation to keywords in the public debate on health care policy.

Regarding the selection of media sources for an analysis of public discourse, the French daily newspaper Le Monde is chosen for several reasons: It has a relatively high circulation—next to Le Figaro (ACPM, 2020), but—as opposed to the comparably prominent newspapers—has a quasi-iconic status (Wilcox, 2005). Moreover, existing research analyzing public discourse selects Le Monde as the French newspaper with reference to its dominance in the coverage of political issues (Jacobs & van Spanje, 2020). Even if the fact that it is a center-left newspaper may imply that reports on political issues are written from a left-wing ideological view, the main idea of the discourse analysis is to trace policy ideas independent of their evaluation or frame back to policy actors. And even if the leftist orientation of the newspaper would result in a bias that grants more presence in newspaper to some policy actors but not others (and some ideas but not others), the multi-methodological procedure applied in this study, which also includes the analysis of policy documents and interviews, provides an ideal setting for cross-checking the empirical results of the media analysis. It thereby would enable the identification of actors that are present in the public discourse, but not in the policy process or vice versa.

As a result of the health care reforms 1990–2010 studied, the period between 1 January 1990 and 31 December 2010 is searched for the relevant keywords of health care reforms. The search is performed via LexisNexis (www.nexisuni.com). Specifically, the keywords "social security/health insurance" (sécurité sociale/assurance maladie) and "health policy" (politique de santé) are used as search terms to locate articles dealing with the public debate on health care reform. For *Le Monde*, these search terms yield 168 hits for the specified study period. The articles are downloaded and transferred to a dataset within the discourse network analysis program DNA. After removing duplicates and articles that do not fit the topic, 84 articles remain in the dataset to be analyzed. The link to the dataset is provided in the appendix.

Once the selected articles are integrated into a dataset, the PAF allows for analysis of their content in light of the assumption that programmatic actors ideationally agree on the content of a policy program and use that program in the struggle for authority in the sector. These connections between policy program elements and actors can be tested using discourse network analyses (Bandelow & Hornung, 2019). This leads to the expectation that indicators of programmatic action are not limited to an observed substantial connection between adopted policies, but also include an assessment that actors who promote these policy programs use the same narrative in the public discourse and share a common view of policy problems and solutions in their sector. Thus, the analysis focuses exclusively on statements that can be directly attributed to individual actors, as the PAF's perspective is on individual actors. However, actors appearing in the discourse network cannot be compared to programmatic actors. Actors that appear in public discourse are mostly politicians and well-known, memorable individuals, while programmatic actors are sectoral actors that do not follow the media or political logic. The discourse network thus presents an initial indication of a unanimously agreed policy program, but without already revealing programmatic actors.

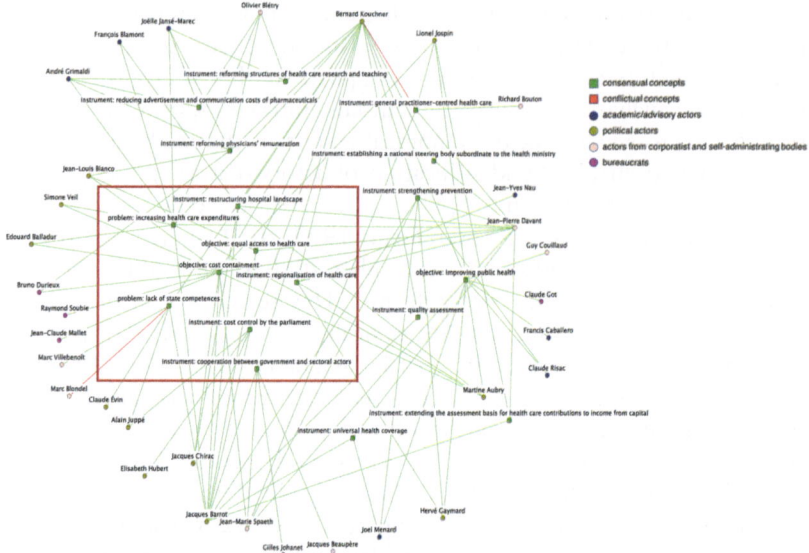

Fig. 5.1 Discourse network of health policy in France, 1990–1999. Source: Own illustration, created with the software visone (Brandes & Wagner, 2019). The red outlines emphasize the programmatic content of the discourse

Figure 5.1 depicts the discourse network resulting from the coding of statements in the selected articles. To allow a comparison of discourse development over time, Fig. 5.1 starts with the discourse network between 1990 and 1999, while Fig. 5.2 presents the discourse network of the second period under study, 2000—2010. The coding procedure is theoretically driven and oriented toward the definition of a policy program as identified problems and corresponding instruments presented as solutions to this problem, as well as the articulation of policy goals (Bandelow et al., 2021; Genieys & Hassenteufel, 2015, p. 282). Thus, the concepts visible in the discourse network are explicitly labeled as problems, solutions, and objectives. To increase the validity of the coding, the procedure was run twice. This results in a final set of 317 coded statements. Not all coded statements are shown in the figures; some actors and concepts were deleted due to redundancy, isolation, or non-specific statements. Since the goal of the discourse networks is to analyze whether actors are connected and which concepts are consensually discussed in the public debate, deleting isolates does not distort the results.

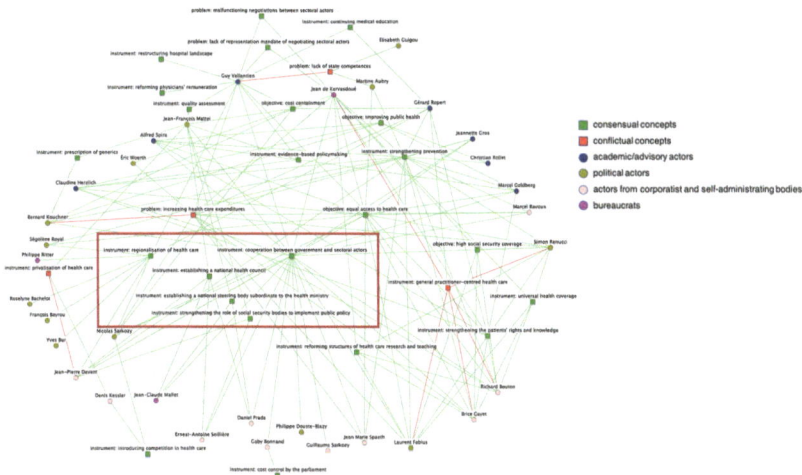

Fig. 5.2 Discourse network of health policy in France, 2000–2010. Source: Own illustration, created with the software visone (Brandes & Wagner, 2019). The red outlines emphasize the programmatic content of the discourse

When interpreting the discourse network, the first thing that stands out is the general agreement present in the newspaper articles and the presence of certain people and concepts that are highly visible in the network. In terms of people, there is considerable visibility of politicians, particularly prime ministers Alain Juppé, Lionel Jospin, and Edouard Balladur, president Jacques Chirac and health ministers Jacques Barrot, Jean-Louis Bianco, Martine Aubry, and to some extent their state secretaries, Hervé Gaymard and Bernard Kouchner. In the PAF's understanding, the latter in particular are to be considered as potential programmatic actors, as they are members of the health care administration. Others, such as Jean-Pierre Davant as president of the National Federation of French Mutualities (Fédération Nationale de la Mutualité Française, FNMF), also actively participated in the discourse and agreed with the concepts presented, but were not members of the narrow state apparatus in the strict sense. With respect to the content of the discourse and the elements of a potential program, it can be postulated that there is both coherence and unanimity regarding the problems identified, the desired objectives, and the preferred instruments to solve these problems and achieve these objectives. In line with what the analysis of adopted policies has indicated above, the identified problems are the increasing health care expenditures, which are associated by some actors with a problem of a lack of state competences to control these expenditures. This gives rise to the objective of cost containment, which is to be achieved through the instruments of increased hierarchical control (by parliament) and various hospital restructurings, modified remuneration and reimbursement systems, the expansion of contribution bases, and the reduction of drug costs, for example, through the prescription of generics. In parallel, there is another dominant goal, which is to achieve equal access to care, leading several actors to call for a universal health coverage, which was actually adopted in 2000.

There is little disagreement on specific concepts, for example, from Marc Blondel, who participated in an employment summit organized in Matignon to bring together sectoral actors and align them with the Plan Juppé (Dive, 2016, p. 108), and who as a leading unionist of the Force Ouvrière (FO) and publicly campaigned against the Plan Juppé (also visible in this network). He complained that he had not been sufficiently involved in the process, while others, including Jean-Marie Spaeth, welcomed the fact that Juppé did not give in to the unions' demands (Bezat & Lemaître, 1997). Despite this disagreement, which was even more present in the articles but not directly linked to identifiable individuals—but to organizations—the problems, objectives, and instruments discussed reflect well the content of the laws previously analyzed. At first glance, this may seem a tautological conclusion—that what is decided is what is talked about publicly—but the discourse network explicitly serves to identify individuals and connect the program to potentially relevant individuals and groups, who are later analyzed with regard to their biographical connections. If these are confirmed, an instance of programmatic action can be assumed. Furthermore, the analysis of media articles along the 1990–2010 timeline also allows for a reconstruction of developments from a long-term perspective:

French health policy at the beginning of the 1990s was characterized by the impression of policy failure, as attempts to decrease health expenditures in previous years had not been successful. The threat of a strike offensive by physicians unwilling to agree to the cost-containment policies favored by the government and the social security system exacerbated the situation. The minister at the time, Jean-Louis Bianco, tried to find a cooperative solution with the physicians' associations and sickness funds, represented by various unions. However, this failed almost completely, as the agreement reached by the sectoral actors did not contribute to the goal of cost containment but, on the contrary, provided for a short-time increase in health care spending. Moreover, the agreement was not accepted by some unions, partly because the representative corporate actor negotiating with the government did not have a representative mandate to conclude binding agreements for all actors. To achieve the common goal of cost containment, various policy solutions were publicly discussed and debated, sometimes supported by reports from expert committees such as the commission chaired by Raymond Soubie. When the first step of the Plan Juppé was communicated through the media, some of the instruments already in place were highlighted, such as the extension of the contribution base to include capital income and increased parliamentary control of health care spending. The experience of previous years prompted actors already occupying key positions to learn from the past and propose new ideas to contain health care costs.

Following a report by IGAS and other institutions, central savings through a restructuring of the hospital landscape were also proposed in 1994 (Blamont, 1994). Regarding the Plan Juppé, pressure from unions and employers' associations was so great in some cases that a move away from the parity system was discussed. This would have been the path to a commercial insurance system. During this period, there were also calls for a national health conference involving all stakeholders to discuss the way forward in terms of cost reduction (and ultimately, probably, also implementation of Plan Juppé). The general discussion was also strongly geared toward bringing the various actors together, which was also foreseen in the Plan Juppé, as it ultimately helped calm some of the public protests. This conference was held for the first time in 1996, also to approve the first of the annual financial laws. The Plan Juppé was adopted in several steps, starting with a constitutional reform and followed by several ordinances.

Despite the fierce opposition from sectoral actors, particularly opposition of physicians' associations to collective liability for exceeding spending targets, and some unions (notably FO), health policy experts such as Jean-Pierre Davant, then head of the French Mutualité, praised the reform for fundamentally restructuring the health care system. Increased oversight of all health care spending was a novum in French health care policy and was therefore frequently discussed. Previous instruments focused largely on controlling reimbursements, but this led to increasing inequality in health care and was detrimental to less affluent citizens. In response to rising claims of inequality in French health care, the 1999 Act Creating the Universal Health Coverage (Couverture Maladie Universelle) (Chauchard & Marié, 2001) under minister Martine Aubry strengthened universal access to health care for all, regardless of social situation. This can also be seen as part of the program of the programmatic group, as it was advocated by the same actors. In an interview with Le Monde, Jacques Barrot, then health minister, paraphrases the policy program, which can best be named "Achieving cost containment by maintaining the main principles of the French health care system".

Particularly present in the media was the strengthened role of parliament in setting the annual budget for health insurance. When the first report of the High Committee on Public Health (which became the High Council on Public Health in 2004 as a result of the Douste-Blazy reform) was published in September 1996, shortly before the first of the annual conferences to prepare the draft legislation for the parliament, the issue of inequality regained attention in the public debate. A case was made for placing the objective of equal access to health care on equal footing with the objective of cost containment. Besides, there was also increased emphasis on the objective of improving public health and strengthening prevention to reduce health care costs. For example, the 1991 Loi Évin restricted advertising for alcohol and tobacco, partly following a European directive, but also partly inspired by the work of professor Claude Got. As an advisor to the health minister, he substantially influenced government policy toward public health. At first glance, this strongly resembles the logic of policy-making from the perspective of the MSF, with a policy entrepreneur advocating a single policy. However, discourse analysis shows that the reference to public health recurs in the discourse, for example, in the reimbursement of specific cancer screenings for women.

After the completion of the Plan Juppé, and thus the first major part of the policy program, the discourse turns from increased state control, parliamentary oversight of spending, universal health coverage, and the extension of contribution bases to include capital income, all of which were still being implemented in the 1990s, to the centralization and regionalization of health care, as already called for in Raymond Soubie's report. These demands also go hand in hand with an aspiration to increase patient participation in health policy, which many policy actors publicly refer to as health democracy (see, e.g., Bernard Kouchner in an interview with *Le Monde* on 28 March 2001). In 1998, a reference doctor system was introduced, in which reimbursements were reduced for patients who did not choose a physician they would consult before seeing another doctor (usually a specialist). This system was replaced by the "treating physician" in 2004 (Barnay et al., 2007). Parliamentary oversight of health care spending, however, did not lead to significant improvements. The ONDAM was missed annually, and physician and hospital strikes led to the health ministry caving in to spend even more money. Despite these negative experiences, there was strong support for the parliamentary oversight of budgets, and thus for a strengthened role for parliament and the state in setting overall health policy guidelines. The problem was clearly in the implementation of these measures. This is where the second period picks up:

In contrast to the discourse network of the first period, this second discourse network appears much denser and more integrated. Initially, this indicates a stronger interconnectedness among health policy actors. Some actors have remained in the public discourse, for example, Jean-Pierre Davant and Bernard Kouchner, while others have joined because they were given important offices, such as Jean-François Mattei as health minister and Nikolas Sarkozy as president. It is also interesting to note that actors who were familiar from the commissions in the early 1990s, including Claudine Herzlich, Christian Rollet, and Jean de Kervasdoué, now entered the public discourse and advanced the instruments they had previously developed. Specifically, the problem of rising health care expenditures remained, but was partly addressed with other instruments, as some instruments had already been implemented (e.g., cost control by parliament). The discourse then evolved in the direction of calling for increased cooperation between the state on the one hand and the regions and corporate actors on the other, often combined with calls for new institutions to be created. In addition, the issue of improving public health gained attention in the public discourse and was often met with calls for strengthening prevention.

The centralization and pooling of competences and the assignment of clear responsibilities to actors of the health care sector became a central concern. The Douste-Blazy reform succeeded in tying corporatist and sectoral actors to health policy governance by merging representative bodies and establishing, for example, the UNCAM as the main representative and steering body of national sickness funds and HAS. These developments culminated with the Plan Hôpital 2007, the preparation of the HPST. It established regional health agencies that were consecutively entrusted with the task of implementing the nationally set targets and objectives at the regional level.

The analysis of media articles, similar to the analysis of legislative texts already carried out, showed that the identified policy program, which was pushed over several years, did not prevent certain policies from being put on the agenda that were not directly linked to the policy program. An example of the non-implementation of proposals that were on the table is the privatization of health care, which was called for in part in conjunction with the introduction of competition in health care. However, these initiatives did not make it into the core of the reform programs.

The networks make it clear that a program becomes entrenched over time as the public shares and openly communicates program's narrative. While the general objectives and identified problems, as well as instruments to address them, remain stable over time, some instruments become more focused than others once the initial reforms are passed. For example, after cost control by parliament was adopted as part of the Plan Juppé, this specific instrument faded from spotlight, while other instruments of state control, such as the regionalization of health care combined with increased responsibility for meeting targets set at the federal level, gained more attention.

This does not mean that all individuals who are in the discourse network are also part of the programmatic group. A true programmatic group can only be identified if, beyond discourse networks, biographical connections between actors who collectively relate to the program are also identified. At the same time, discourse networks show that public media coverage is often dominated by certain types of actors, including primarily journalists, academics, and politicians. While public discourse reflects the narratives found in policy proposals and intellectual documents and reports, it is clear that it is political rather than administrative actors who appear in newspapers. This is partly because administrative actors largely operate behind the scenes and follow a different logic than politicians, whose primary goals include seeking office and votes.

Consequently, politicians also use media attention to gain exposure among their constituents and attract potential voters. In terms of the PAF, it becomes visible that the promotion of a particular policy program, which may also be associated with a programmatic group hidden from media attention, may well lead to appointment as a minister. Thus, politicians can be part of programmatic groups and use policy programs to gain offices in key positions of government. Interestingly, a discourse network analysis also reveals the possibility that some politicians may publicly change their minds on certain issues in response to polls and approval of a policy among actors in the policy process. Hence, a discourse network analysis of a public media discourse provides a small but important aspect to the larger picture of a programmatic group behind the publicly discussed policy program. To gain deeper insight into the formal roles and networks of potential programmatic actors, it is essential to look more closely at the formal and informal actor positions that play a role in policy-making and the biographical connections that link them.

5.3   Biographies and Identities of French Programmatic Actors

Formally, Dominique Libault clearly occupies a central position as director of the DSS between 2002 and 2012, when both the Douste-Blazy reform and the HPST were adopted. He replaced Pierre-Louis Bras, who had headed this directorate for the previous two years but had been a central adviser in the cabinets of Claude Évin (1988–1991) and Martine Aubry (Le Monde, 2000). Before Bras, Raoul Briet had headed the directorate, and he had served on the Soubie Commission, which elaborated the health policy program. The divisions of the health ministry thus emerge as a central—and formal—position of power where programs are elaborated and programmatic actors sit.

Besides the formally important health ministry, the overview of the French health care system (Fig. 4.1) identified other institutions that are directly involved in the decision-making processes of French health policy. One of these is the representative body of the sickness funds, UNCAM. Since UNCAM was only founded in 2004, it makes sense to include the National Health Insurance Fund (Caisse Nationale de l'Assurance Maladie; CNAM) in this sample as well. The other institutions identified as formally relevant to the decision-making processes of French health policy according to Fig. 4.1 include the IGAS, the HAS, the HCAAM, and the CNS, some of which were created as recently as the early 2000s. Given that the creation of new institutions can be seen as a key element in the long-term stability of a policy program, a closer look at these institutions can also shed light on the actors who then occupied leading positions in these bodies based on their affiliation with a programmatic group. The formal analysis here starts from a thorough overview of who the actors were who occupied these positions between 1990 and 2010.

Table 5.2 lists the respective individuals occupying key positions in these institutions. Regarding the CNS, due to its more than 72 members over the years in the period studied, it is difficult to provide a concise

Table 5.2 Occupied positions in key institutions of French health policy

Name	Time	Position
DSS (Direction de la Sécurité Sociale/Directorate of Social Security)		
Rollande Ruellan	1994–1996	Director
Raoul Briet	1996–2000	Director
Pierre-Louis Bras	2000–2002	Director
Dominique Libault	2002–2012	Director
Thomas Fatome	2012–2017	Director
Mathilde Lignot-Leloup	2017–2020	Director
Franck von Lennep	Since 2020	Director
UNCAM (Union Nationale des Caisses d'Assurance Maladie/National Union of Health Insurance Funds, founded in 2004)		
Michel Régereau	2004–2014	Président du Conseil
William Gardey	2014–2019	President du Conseil
Fabrice Gombert	Since 2020	President du Conseil
Frédéric Van Roekeghem	2004–2014	General Director
Nicolas Revel	2014–2020	General Director
Thomas Fatome	Since 2020	General Director
IGAS (Inspection Générale des Affaires Sociales/General Inspectorate of Social Affairs, founded in 1967)		
Michel Lucas	1982–1993	General Director
Christian Rollet	1993–2000	General Director
Marie-Caroline Bonnet-Galzy	2000–2006	General Director
André Nutte	2006–2009	General Director
Pierre Boissier	2009–2017	General Director
Nathalie Destais	Since 2017	General Director
HCAAM (Haut Conseil pour l'Avenir de l'Assurance maladie/High Council for the Future of Health Insurance, founded in 2003)		
Anne-Marie Brocas	Since 2003	President
Pierre-Jean Lancry	Since 2003	Vice President
HAS (Haute Autorité de santé/High Authority for Health, founded in 2004)		
Laurent Degos	2005–2010	President
Raoul Briet	2004–2010	Member of college
Jean-Paul Guérin	2004–2014	Member of college
Bernard Guiraud-Chaumeil	2004–2008	Member of college
Pascale Briand	2004–2006	Member of college
Gilles Bouvenot	2004–2014	Member of college
Étienne Caniard	2004–2010	Member of college
Claude Maffioli	2004–2010	Member of college
Lise Rochaix	2006–2014	Member of college
Jean-Michel Dubernard	Since 2008	Member of college
Cédric Grouchka	Since 2010	Member of college
Jean-Luc Harousseau	2011–2016	President
Alain Cordier	2011–2018	Member of college
Jean-François Thebaut	2011–2016	Member of college

(*continued*)

Table 5.2 (continued)

Name	Time	Position
Yvonnick Morice	2014–2020	Member of college
Jacques Belghiti	2014–2020	Member of college
Loïc Guillevin	2014–2020	Member of college
Agnès Buzyn	2016–2017	President
Isabelle Adenot	Since 2017	Member of college
Anne-Marie Armanteras-de Saxcé	2017–2020	Member of college
Elisabeth Bouvet	Since 2017	Member of college
Christian Saout	Since 2017	Member of college
Christian Thuillez	Since 2017	Member of college
Dominique Le Guludec	Since 2017	President
Catherine Geindre	Since 2020	Member of college
Valérie Paris	Since 2020	Member of college
Pierre Cochat	Since 2020	Member of college

Source: Société Générale de Presse (2020)

representation of members. Moreover, the CNS is not a formal professional position, but rather it is the professional position that leads to participation in the CNS. Thus, it is an indicator rather than a manifestation of relevant individuals. In addition, the legal basis of the CNS has changed substantially, with the creation of regional health councils in 2002 and a new CNS with a larger number of members in 2005. Nevertheless, the annual compositions have been scanned (Brodin, 2000, 2001; de Paillerets, 1999; Menard, 1996) and selected individuals are presented as examples to substantiate their role in French health policy because of their involvement in the public discourse and the CNS. For example, Richard Bouton (with 11 statements) and Joël Menard (with 3 statements) were already visible in the discourse networks and active in the public debate, and both participated in the first national health conference in 1996; Menard even chaired it (Menard, 1996). Richard Bouton occupies a central position as president of a physicians' association, the French Federation of General Practitioners (Fédération Française des Médecins Généralistes, MG). Joël Menard was included as a professional expert. Other experts included in the CNS and also visible in the discourse network were Alfred Spira and Jean-Marie Bertrand, who was explicitly requested as an expert for the drafting of the HPST law (Secrétariat de la Conférence Nationale de Santé, 2010, p. 21).

According to the PAF research protocol, the analysis of professional actor biographies proceeds starts from the analysis of formal and informal actor positions. The first step was to identify all individuals who held these positions during the period under study. The second step is to analyze who the "long-timers" (Darviche et al., 2013) in these positions are, not in the sense that they have occupied the same position for several years, but that they have made their career in the health care system. Once these individuals have been identified, a more detailed analysis looks at their individual biographical files. This allows both a revelation of individual careers as targets of programmatic action and of biographical intersections as roots of programmatic action.

In French health policy between 1990 and 2010, several of the actors originally involved in generating and promoting the ideas that were later translated into policy actually climbed the career ladder. Referring directly to the members of the commissions mentioned in Sect. 5.1, Raymond Soubie himself became social policy advisor to president Sarkozy until 2010. His was succeeded by Jean Castex, who had previously been head of Xavier Bertrand's cabinet, former health minister (2006–2007), and labor minister (2007–2008), and even made it to prime minister in 2020 (Ficek & Godeluck, 2020). Raoul Briet, who had already been a member of the Soubie Commission, became director of the National Old-Age Insurance Fund for Salaried Employees (Caisse nationale d'assurance-vieillesse des travailleurs salaries; CNAVTS) immediately after the report was published (Juillard, 1994). Two years later, he was promoted to director of the social security (directeur de la sécurité sociale), and in 2012, he became president of the first chamber of the Cours des Comptes (Court of Auditors), one of the most important institutions in the French administrative system (Cour des Comptes, 2020). His key role in the Plan Juppé has also been reflected in media reports (Bezat & Lemaître, 1997).

Apart from the DSS, the discourse network has uncovered some actors of the Soubie Commission who remained or returned to the public spotlight, including Claudine Herzlich, Christian Rollet, and Jean de Kervasdoué. Jean de Kervasdoué and the then director of the CNAM, Gilles Johanet, were also associated with the program developed in the Soubie Commission (Hassenteufel, 2008). Other commissions formed, for example, for the preparation of the HPST, which was mainly inspired by a commission chaired by Gérard Larcher, had as advisors Edouard Couty, Jean-Pierre Davant, Jean de Kervasdoué, and Guy Vallancien (Ministère des Solidarités et de la Santé, 2008), who were already active in the discourse network.

In order to outline how the biographies of actors coincide, and to use this as a further indication of the presence of programmatic action as revealed step by step in the previous steps, the following biographies serve as anchoring examples. They were selected either because of their occupation of formal power positions or because of their appearance in the media as a result of their participation in the Soubie Commission. The source of all biographical files is the biographical database of the Société Générale de Presse (2020).

Anchoring Example: Pierre-Louis Bras (selected positions)
- *1982–1984* Student at the National School of Administration l'Ecole Nationale d'Administration, ENA)
- *1988–1991* Policy officer in the office of the Minister of Solidarity, Health and Social Protection (Claude Evin)
- *1991–1993* Director of the cabinet of the general budget rapporteur at the National Assembly (Alain Richard)
- *1993–1994* General Manager of the Mutualité de la fonction publique (Civil Service Mutual Insurance)
- *1994–1997* Director of the local authority market at Société Générale
- *1997–2000* Adviser in charge of social protection in the office of the Minister of Employment and Solidarity (Martine Aubry)
- *2000* Deputy Director of the Private Office of the Minister for Employment and Solidarity (Martine Aubry), responsible for Social Security, Social Protection and Health
- *2000–2002* Director of Social Security at the Ministry of Employment and Solidarity then (May 2002) under the joint authority of the Ministry of Social Affairs, Labour and Solidarity and the Minister of Health, Family and Disabled Persons
- *Since 2003* Inspector General of Social Affairs (external tower)
- *Since 2015* Chairman of the Pension Guidance Council, Prime Minister's Office
- *Since 2015* Chairman of the steering committee of the technical agency for information on hospitalization

Anchoring Example: Anne-Marie Brocas (selected positions)
- *1980–1982* Student at the National School of Administration l'Ecole Nationale d'Administration, ENA)
- *1990–1991* Technical Advisor to the Office of the Minister Delegate for Health (Bruno Durieux)

- *1991–1992* Deputy Director of the Office of the Minister Delegate for Health (Bruno Durieux)
- *1992–1994* Deputy Director of Health Insurance in the Social Security Directorate of the Ministry of Health
- *1992*: Chairwoman of the Workshop "Financial Perspectives of the Health System" held at the Commissariat au Plan within the framework of the health system prospective group
- *1994–2000* Head of department, assistant to the director of social security, at the Ministry of Social Affairs, Health and Urban Affairs
- *1999* in charge of the coordination of the Etats Généraux de la Santé (General Health Assembly)
- *1999* General Rapporteur of the Social Europe Group at the French Planning Commission (Commissariat au Plan)
- *2006–2012* Director of Research, Studies, Evaluation and Statistics on Health and Solidarity, under the joint authority of the Ministry of Labour, Employment and Health and the Ministry of the Budget, Public Accounts and State Reform
- *Since 2012* Inspector General of Social Affairs (appointed on 1 September 2013)
- *Since 2014* President of the High Council for the Future of Health Insurance (HCAAM)

Anchoring Example: Dominique Libault (selected positions)
- *1985–1987* Student at the National School of Administration l'Ecole Nationale
- *1987* Second class civil administrator, assigned to the Ministry of Social Affairs and Employment. Head of the Office Al-Scope, Contributions, Other Receipts—at the Sub-Directorate for Administrative and Financial Affairs of the Social Security Directorate
- *1993–1995* Secretary general of the conseil supérieur de la mutualité
- *1993–1995* Technical adviser in the office of the Minister of State, Minister of Social Affairs, Health and Urban Affairs (Simone Veil)
- *1995* Sub-Director of Access to Care, Social Security Directorate, Ministry of Solidarity between Generations
- *1995–2000* Deputy Director of Social Security Financing and Management in the Social Security Directorate, Ministry of Employment and Solidarity
- *1999* Reappointed Director, representing the Minister for Social Security, of the Caisse d'amortissement de la dette sociale (CADES)

- *2000–2002* Head of Department, Deputy Director of Social Security, at the Ministry of Employment and Solidarity, then (May 2002) under the joint authority of the Ministry of Social Affairs, Labour and Solidarity and the Ministry of Health, Family and the Disabled
- *2002–2012* Director of social security, under the joint authority of the Ministry of Labour, Employment and Health and the Ministry of the Budget, Public Accounts and State Reform
- *Since 2012* State Councilor (external tour)
- *Since 2012* Vice-Chairman of the High Council on the Financing of Social Protection
- *Since 2012* Director General of the Ecole Nationale Supérieure de Sécurité Sociale (EN3S)

Anchoring Example: Didier Tabuteau (selected positions)
- *1982–1984*   Student at the National School of Administration l'Ecole Nationale d'Administration, ENA)
- *1985–1987* Student at the National School of Administration l'Ecole Nationale d'Administration, ENA)
- *1988–1991* Technical adviser in the office of the Minister of National Solidarity, Health and Social Protection (Claude Evin)
- *1992–1993* Director of the Cabinet of the Minister of Health and Humanitarian Action (Bernard Kouchner)
- *1997–2000* Deputy Director of the Office of the Minister for Employment and Solidarity (Martine Aubry)
- *Since 1999* State Councilor
- *2000* Adviser to the Minister for Employment and Solidarity (Martine Aubry), in charge of preparing the bill on patients' rights and the modernization of the health system
- *2001–2002* Director of the Office of the Minister Delegate for Health (Bernard Kouchner)
- *2008–2012* Director of the Centre d'analyse des politiques publiques en santé, Ecole des hautes études de santé publique (EHESP)
- *Since 2017* Deputy president of the social section at the Council of State

Whether the biographies of actors associated with the policy program actually overlap and can be traced back to common working occasions is best assessed when tracing them back to commissions like the Soubie Commission, which presents a central starting point for programmatic actors who later occupied key positions in various newly created agencies. The members, including above all Raoul Briet, Anne-Marie Brocas, Jean de Kervasdoué, and Raymond Soubie, subsequently held central positions that were central in the further course of French health policy. This applies, for example, to the Larcher Commission, but also to the DSS in the Ministry of Health, which was significantly strengthened in its competencies by the reforms of the policy program. It can thus be seen here that the actors, who are biographically linked to each other, have themselves attained positions that they have strengthened through their own program. The further biographical connections here also show a strong network between the central actors in health policy, who were also already present in the discourse network and were repeatedly mentioned as essential figures in the political process.

5.4   Continuous Programmatic Action in French Health Policy After the Financial Crisis

Looking more closely at the period after 2010 (see Table 5.3), both with regard to the content of health care reforms and the actors involved, we can see that the programmatic group was active during that period as well. With regard to health care reforms, the legislation through 2013 adjusted measures that had already been passed, such as the HPST act. In 2011, regulations on the use of medicines not yet approved were tightened and a new agency was created, the National Agency of Medicine and Health Products Safety (Agence nationale de sécurité du médicament et des produits de santé; ANSM). These policies followed the scandal around the Mediator drug, which was prescribed for patients suffering from diabetes and obesity but apparently caused up to 2000 deaths because it had not been banned by the responsible French agency following indications of questionable value and scientific evidence for its safety (Mullard, 2011), and another such quality-related incident involving breast implants (Emmerich et al., 2012; Lochouarn, 2012).

In 2013, a national health strategy was announced by then health minister Marisol Touraine to guide the health reforms under the label of reducing inequality, strengthening regional and local initiatives including ARSs and primary care, and overall increasing the efficiency of the health care system (Touraine, 2014). In her major reform to modernize the health system in 2016, the trend toward territorialization, which had been inherent since the Plan Juppé, is further reinforced. The law creates

Table 5.3 Substantial health care reforms in France 2010–2020

Designation of reforms	Main reform content
LOI n° 2011-940 du 10 août 2011 modifiant certaines dispositions de la loi n° 2009-879 du 21 juillet 2009 portant réforme de l'hôpital et relative aux patients, à la santé et aux territoires	Abolishes the financial penalties (up to 3000 euros per year) applicable to general practitioners in overcrowded areas refusing to contribute to the provision of care in undercrowded areas, maintaining the obligation for doctors to declare their planned absences in advance to the departmental council of the order, requiring practitioners to provide their patients with detailed information on the purchase price of prostheses and appliances
LOI n° 2011-2012 du 29 décembre 2011 relative au renforcement de la sécurité sanitaire du médicament et des produits de santé	Following the Mediator scandal, the reform concentrates on health safety and therapeutic progress and introduces more strict guidelines on the transparency of health authorities' decisions and links of interest. The Temporary Use Authorization (autorisations temporaires d'utilisation (ATU) enabling the use of medicinal products without formal market admission. The law enforces these regulations, and creates a new agency, the National Agency of Medicine and Health Products Safety (Agence nationale de sécurité du médicament et des produits de santé; ANSM)
LOI n° 2014-57 du 27 janvier 2014 relative aux modalités de mise en œuvre des conventions conclues entre les organismes d'assurance maladie complémentaire et les professionnels, établissements et services de santé (1)	Obliges the government to submit to Parliament an annual report drawing up an assessment and evaluation of the agreements mentioned in Article L. 863-8 of the Social Security Code. The report shall focus in particular on the guarantees and benefits that these agreements provide, their consequences for patients, particularly in terms of access to care and the amount they have to pay, and their impact on the rates and prices charged by the professionals, establishments and services concerned
LOI n° 2016-41 du 26 janvier 2016 de modernisation de notre système de santé (1)	promotes prevention for the fight against tobacco and alcohol, facilitates access to care by a national program to combat medical deserts, establishment of a national telephone number to reach a doctor outside the opening hours of doctors' offices; extension of a social tariff for dental care (dentures and orthodontics), optical (glasses) and hearing aids for beneficiaries of the ACS (aid for the purchase of complementary health care), creation of class actions for victims of damage caused by health products; creates regional hospital groups (GHT) to allow nearby hospitals to share tasks or support functions in a joint medical project, establishment of a territorial health service for the public in five areas: Community Care, Continuity of Care, Prevention, Mental Health and Access to Care for the Disabled; Re-launch of the Common Medical Record, freely accessible to the patient, improves access to health data while respecting privacy

(*continued*)

Table 5.3 (continued)

Designation of reforms	Main reform content
LOI n° 2019-733 du 14 juillet 2019 relative au droit de résiliation sans frais de contrats de complémentaire santé (1)	Charges the National Union of Supplementary Health Insurance Organisations with monitoring the effective implementation by supplementary health insurance organizations of digital services enabling their members, insured persons and participants to be aware of their rights and guarantees in real time and making it possible for professionals, establishments, and health centers to be provided with information relating to these rights and guarantees
LOI n° 2019-774 du 24 juillet 2019 relative à l'organisation et à la transformation du système de santé (1)	Removes the numerus clausus determining access to the second year of undergraduate studies, the number of students trained in medicine, pharmacy, dentistry, and midwifery will be determined within the framework of regulatory procedures, taking into account training capacities and the needs of the health system, and based on consultation between the universities and the regional health agencies. Developing a collective care system, between professionals and the ambulatory, medico-social, or hospital sector, and to better structure the supply of care in the territories. It encourages the development of regional health projects. Creating the territorial health project, which will give concrete expression to the objective of decompartmentalizing the city, hospital, and medico-social sectors. Stipulating that the projects of the territorial professional health communities (CPTS) will be submitted for approval to the director general of the regional health agency in order to ensure their coordination with the other players in the health system. In the CPTS, all health professionals will have to work in a network. Creation of a new data platform. Expanding possibilities of deployment of telemedicine and telecare by adjusting the legal framework

Source: République Française (2020)

regional hospital groups (groupements hospitaliers de territoire, GHT) to replace CHTs. Since the latter were formed on a voluntary basis and the GHTs are mandatory entities that must work closely with the ARSs to ensure access to health care across the landscape, this is a new form of territorial organization of health care in medical deserts (Tourmente, 2016). The path of territorialization taken, which began with the creation of ARSs, thus gained relevance in the 2010s. The 2016 law also introduced the possibility for physicians to register as territorial practitioners, which granted them financial benefits and allowed for special contracts with physicians who chose to work in underserved areas (Hassenteufel et al., 2020, p. 49).

This path of territorialization continues after 2016. The national health strategy "Ma Santé 2022" (My Health 2022) (République Française, 2018) elaborated further programmatic measures, some of which have already been translated into concrete reforms. For example, the 2019 reform on the organization and transformation of the health care system strengthened the role of the ARSs in determining the number of students trained in medical professions, taking into account local needs. It also required the ARS to approve territorial professional health communities (communautés professionnelles territoriales de santé (CPTS)) projects and explicitly promoted regional health projects aimed at increasing efficiency (and thus reducing costs) in the organization of local health care.

Another large part of the ongoing policy program concerns digitalization. The Douste-Blazy reform in 2004 already created a digital health space for patients in the form of a digital health record. This was further extended and access was made easier in the 2019 reform mentioned above. The same reform also expanded telecare and telemedicine capabilities, as well as the storage of health data to improve research. It is likely that the COVID-19 pandemic will initiate further steps toward digitalized health care.

The analysis of the actors connected to these reforms via a discourse network analysis yields mixed results. In general, the coverage of the health political discourse ebbed away in the 2010s, which is why the results of the media analysis are only reported, but not visualized. Looking at the actors publicly referred to in *Le Monde*, the debate centered mainly around political elites, such as the presidents Emmanuel Macron and François Hollande, and the health minister Marisol Touraine. However, Dominique Libault also appeared in the media in 2020 and is thus a sign for continued influence of the programmatic group.

With regard to the content of the discourse, the financial crisis worsened the financial situation of French health policy, which was communicated publicly. Health expenditures rose again and the contribution-financed health care system suffered from a decrease in revenue due to increased unemployment. The introduction of remuneration for general practitioners based on public health objectives (Rémunération sur Objectifs de

Santé Publique; ROSP) has led to an increase in the general practitioners' payment. Nevertheless, they went on strike on the occasion of the health care reform by Marisol Touraine in 2012/2013, because the principle of reimbursement should be replaced by the principle of payment in kind (tiers payant). Her 2016 reform modernized the health care sector by strengthening the information given to patients, introducing a central phone number for patients to receive medical care, and further improving regional health care by following the reform path previously taken in the direction of the ARSs (Casassus, 2015).

In 2018, the care of elderly people moved in the focus of attention as the consent of old-aged persons to be housed in care homes varied. The ethics committee and policy advisors suggested the introduction of a fifth branch of social security, which to that point had not yet been established. In 2020, surprisingly, the outbreak of COVID-19 and the following pandemic dominated the public discourse. It shed light on the problems of the health care system, including the missing focus on public health, and the low salaries that employees in system-relevant professions gained. Several measures were adopted to fight the consequences of the pandemic and to contain the infection dynamics in France. These had been summarized under the label of the Ségur de la santé, but criticized with regard to their lacking consideration of the territorial specificities of health care provision—particularly the hospital landscape—and concerns. The increased turn to a territorialized health policy with the ARSs implementing the nationally set centralized guidelines (and budgets) has furthermore proved less promising than initially thought. The ARSs are said to have not enough competences—above all regarding the control of budgetary means—to ensure a territorially appropriate health care, and are limited in their actions to research, innovation, employment, and training.

Although the discourse analysis of French health policy in 2010–2020 reveals a less dense public debate compared to the previous two decades, the content of the policy program and the actors involved continue to have a major impact on health care reforms. In describing the key evolution in the governance of social security, programmatic actor Dominique Libault points to three key elements of the restructuring of French health policy. In addition to financial oversight of the budget by parliament, and the changing relations between the national and local levels and between state and social security actors, he proposes the creation of councils to guide the future of health policy by bringing together experts, social partners, and members of the administration (Libault & Minonzio, 2015). The establishment of such councils to give direction to health policy allows for the combination of expertise with sectoral and political-administrative actors, ensuring a long-term strategy of health policy for a programmatic group.

With respect to the biographical actor networks, it can also be noted that programmatic action lives on in France. The HAS serves as a source of personnel for higher positions in government and administration, as in the case of Alain Cordier, who was appointed as a special advisor to Christophe Devys, the director general of the ARS in Paris (ARS Île de France, 2018). Anne-Marie Armanteras-de Saxcé becomes an advisor in the president's bureau (Hospimedia, 2020). Figure 5.1 shows how the existing network of programmatic actors has expanded to include other agencies. The origin of this network remains the Soubie Commission. It visualizes how the programmatic group has used the newly created structures to place its members in these power positions and manifest its influence and ideas in these institutional structures. Today's key players, such as Thomas Fatome and Nicolas Revel, as well as Jean Castex and Franck van Lennep, have risen through the old network structures to take the places of Dominique Libault, Pierre-Louis Bras, and Raoul Briet. They are still interconnected through the very institutions through which they gained influence. This network is also created on the basis of the qualitative findings from the interviews, just as the nodes between the core group are depicted based on this information.

The COVID-19 pandemic has not just dominated the media discourse of French health policy, it has also affected the actor networks in the health sector. Responses toward the Corona crisis had been in the French tradition of centralized measures, yet at first without a substantial consideration of regional specificities given that the ARSs are basically implementing national measures at a local level. With increasing turn to decentralized crisis management, COVID-19 can be seen as an accelerator of the previously taken paths toward territorialization and adaptation of measures to local settings, an endeavor in which the programmatic group is ever more visible (Hassenteufel, 2020).

REFERENCES

ACPM, A. p. 1. C. d. 1. P. e. d. M. (2020). Ranking der auflagenstärksten überregionalen Tageszeitungen in Frankreich im Jahr 2019. *https://de.statista.com/statistik/daten/studie/1013180/umfrage/verkaufte-auflage-der-ueberregionalen-tageszeitungen-in-frankreich/ (last retrieved from 5 August 2020)*.

ARS Île de France. (2018). Alain Cordier Nommé Conseiller Spécial du Directeur Général de l'ARS. *https://www.iledefrance.ars.sante.fr/alain-cordier-nomme-conseiller-special-du-directeur-general-de-lars (last retrieved from 27 December 2020)*.

Bandelow, N. C., & Hornung, J. (2019). One Discourse to Rule Them All? Narrating the Agenda for Labor Market Policies in France and Germany. *Policy and Society, 38*(3), 408–428. https://doi.org/10.1080/14494035.2019.1641379

Bandelow, N. C., Hornung, J., & Smyrl, M. (2021). Theoretical Foundations of the Programmatic Action Framework (PAF). *European Policy Analysis, 7*(1), 14–27. https://doi.org/10.1002/epa2.1083

Barnay, T., Hartmann, L., & Ulmann, P. (2007). Réforme du « Médecin traitant » et Nouveaux Enjeux de la Médecine de Ville en France. *Revue française des affaires sociales, 1*, 109–126. https://doi.org/10.3917/rfas.071.0109

Bezat, J.-M. (1993). Le Plan préconise une importante régionalisation du système de santé. *Les Echos https://www.lesechos.fr/1993/07/le-plan-preconise-une-importante-regionalisation-du-systeme-de-sante-908009 (last retrieved from 9 July 2020)*.

Bezat, J.-M., & Lemaître, F. (1997). Comment Alain Juppé, en Voulant Réformer la Sécurité Sociale et les Retraites, Déclencha le Mouvement de l'Automne 1995. *Le Monde. https://www.lemonde.fr/archives/article/1997/05/17/comment-alain-juppe-en-voulant-reformer-la-securite-sociale-et-les-retraites-declencha-le-mouvement-de-l-automne-1995_3755785_1819218.html (last retrieved from 19 October 2020)*.

Blamont, F. (1994). Perspectives. La Croissance des Dépenses de Santé. Les Hôpitaux Publics Sous Pression. Point de Vue. Entre les Mains de Bercy. *Le Monde https://www.lemonde.fr/archives/article/1994/11/01/perspectives-la-croissance-des-depenses-de-sante-les-hopitaux-publics-sous-pression-point-de-vue-entre-les-mains-de-bercy_3848192_1819218.html (last retrieved from 7 October 2020)*.

Bosch, X. (2004). French Government Approves Unpopular Health Reforms. *The Lancet, 363*(9427), 2148. https://doi.org/10.1016/S0140-6736(04)16541-0

Bouget, D. (1998). The Juppé Plan and the Future of the French Social Welfare System. *Journal of European Social Policy, 8*(2), 155–172. https://doi.org/10.1177/095892879800800204

Brandes, U., & Wagner, D. (2019). visone. visual social networks. *http://visone.ethz.ch.*

Bras, P.-L., & Tabuteau, D. (2009). "Santé 2010", un rapport de référence pour les politiques de santé. *Les Tribunes de la santé, 25*(4), 79–93. https://doi.org/10.3917/seve.025.0079

Brodin, M. (2000). Rapport de la Conférence Nationale de Santé—2000. *https://www.vie-publique.fr/sites/default/files/rapport/pdf/004001483.pdf (last retrieved from 19 October 2020).*

Brodin, M. (2001). Rapport de la Conférence Nationale de Santé—2001. *https://www.vie-publique.fr/sites/default/files/rapport/pdf/014000552.pdf (last retrieved from 19 October 2020).*

Capano, G., Howlett, M., Jarvis, D. S. L., Ramesh, M., & Goyal, N. (2020). Mobilizing Policy (In)Capacity to Fight COVID-19: Understanding Variations in State Responses. *Policy and Society, 1-24,* 1. https://doi.org/10.1080/14494035.2020.1787628

Casassus, B. (2015). French Health Workers Strike Over Payment Plan in Health Bill. *The Lancet, 385*(9971), e18. https://doi.org/10.1016/S0140-6736(15)60489-5

Chauchard, J.-P., & Marié, R. (2001). La couverture maladie universelle : résurgence de l'aide sociale ou mutation de la sécurité sociale ? *Revue française des affaires sociales, 4,* 137–156. https://doi.org/10.3917/rfas.014.0137

Cour des Comptes, C. r. t. d. c. (2020). Raoul Briet. *https://www.ccomptes.fr/fr/raoul-briet (last retrieved from 9 July 2020).*

Darviche, M.-S., Genieys, W., Hoeffler, C., & Joana, J. (2013). Des « Long Timers » au Sommet de l'État Américain. *Gouvernement et action publique, 1*(1). https://doi.org/10.3917/gap.131.0007

de Paillerets, F. (1999). Rapport de la Conférence Nationale de Santé—1999. *https://www.vie-publique.fr/sites/default/files/rapport/pdf/004000915.pdf (last retrieved from 19 October 2020).*

Dive, B. (2016). *Alain Juppé. L'Homme Qui Revient de Loin.* L'Archipel.

Emmerich, J., Dumarcet, N., & Lorence, A. (2012). France's New Framework for Regulating Off-Label Drug Use. *New England Journal of Medicine, 367*(14), 1279–1281. https://doi.org/10.1056/NEJMp1208347

Evin, C. (2019). 10 Ans d'ARS : Quel Bilan d'une Forme de Déconcentration Régionale ? *Regards, 56*(2), 105–116. https://doi.org/10.3917/regar.056.0105

Ficek, I., & Godeluck, S. (2020). Remaniement : Jean Castex, le « M. Déconfinement », promu à Matignon. *Les Echos https://www.lesechos.fr/politique-societe/gouvernement/portrait-jean-castex-le-m-deconfinement-promu-a-matignon-1221049 (last retrieved from 9 July 2020).*

Genieys, W., & Hassenteufel, P. (2001). Entre les politiques publiques et la politique: l'émergence d'une "élite du Welfare"? *Revue française des affaires sociales, 4*(4), 41–50.

Genieys, W., & Hassenteufel, P. (2015). The Shaping of New State Elites: Healthcare Policymaking in France Since 1981. *Comparative Politics, 47*(3), 280–295. Retrieved from http://www.jstor.org/stable/43664147

Grimaldi, A. (2015). Si la loi HPST m'était contée.... *Les Tribunes de la santé, 46*(1), 57–63. https://doi.org/10.3917/seve.046.0057

Hassenteufel, P. (2008). L'évolution des rapports de pouvoirs dans un système bismarckien: le cas de la France. *Santé, Société et Solidarité, 2008*(2), 63–70.

Hassenteufel, P. (2012). Les Sources Intellectuelles des Réformes du Système de Santé Francais: La Prédominance des Forums et des Acteurs Administratifs. In J. De Kervasdoué (Ed.), *Carnet de Santé de la France*. Economica.

Hassenteufel, P. (2020). Handling the COVID-19 Crisis in France: Politicization and Policy Changes in a Centralized State-led Health System. *European Policy Analysis, 6*(2), 1.

Hassenteufel, P., & Palier, B. (2005). Les Trompe-l'œil de la « Gouvernance » de l'Assurance Maladie. *Revue Française d'Administration Publique, 113*(1), 13–27. https://doi.org/10.3917/rfap.113.0013

Hassenteufel, P., & Palier, B. (2016). The French Welfare System. In R. Elgie, E. Grossman, & A. G. Mazur (Eds.), *The Oxford Handbook of French Politics* (pp. 60–78). Oxford University Press.

Hassenteufel, P., Schweyer, F.-X., Gerlinger, T., Henkel, R., Lückenbach, C., & Reiter, R. (2020). The Role of Professional Groups in Policy Change: Physician's Organizations and the Issue of Local Medical Provision Shortages in France and Germany. *European Policy Analysis, 6*(1), 38–57. https://doi.org/10.1002/epa2.1073

Hassenteufel, P., Smyrl, M., Genieys, W., & Moreno-Fuentes, F. J. (2010). Programmatic Actors and the Transformation of European Health Care States. *Journal of Health Politics, Policy and Law, 35*(4), 517–538. https://doi.org/1 0.1215/03616878-2010-015

Hospimedia, L. a. d. t. d. s. (2020). Politique de santé: Anne-Marie Armanteras-de Saxcé rejoint l'Élysée sur la santé, le grand âge et le handicap. *https://www. hospimedia.fr/actualite/nominations/20200228-politique-de-sante-anne-marie-armanteras-de-saxce (last retrieved from 27 December 2020)*.

IRDES, I. d. R. e. D. e. É. d. l. S. (2018). Loi Hôpital Patients Santé et Territoires. Synthèse Documentaire. *https://www.irdes.fr/documentation/syntheses/loi-bachelot-hopital-patients-sante-et-territoires-hpst.pdf (last retrieved from 21 August 2020)*.

Jacobs, L., & van Spanje, J. (2020). Prosecuted, Yet Popular? Hate Speech Prosecution of Anti-immigration Politicians in the News and Electoral Support.

Comparative European Politics. doi:https://doi.org/10.1057/s41295-020-00215-4

Juillard, L.-E. (1994). Raoul Briet, un professionnel du social à la tête de la CNAVTS. *Les Echos https://www.lesechos.fr/1994/02/raoul-briet-un-profes sionnel-du-social-a-la-tete-de-la-cnavts-1042215 (last retrieved from 9 July 2020).*

Lancry, P.-J., & Sandier, S. (1999). Rationing Health Care in France. *Health Policy, 50*(1), 23–38. https://doi.org/10.1016/S0168-8510(99)00062-7

Le Monde, F. (2000). Emploi et Solidarité. *Le Monde https://www.lemonde.fr/ archives/article/2000/07/29/emploi-et-solidarite_3611313_1819218.html (last retrieved from 7 October 2020).*

Libault, D., & Minonzio, J. (2015). La Transformation du Pilotage de la Sécurité Sociale : une Expérience Pour l'eÉnsemble de l'Action Publique. Entretien avec Dominique Libault, Propos recueillis par Jérôme Minonzio. *Informations sociales, 189*(3), 72–79. https://doi.org/10.3917/inso.pre.0072

Lochouarn, M. (2012). France Launches New Drug Regulatory Agency. *The Lancet, 379*(9832), 2136. https://doi.org/10.1016/S0140-6736(12)60927-1

Lopez, A. (2010). Les Agences Régionales de Santé (ARS), une Question d'Équilibres Entre des Objectifs Différents et des Mécanismes de Régulation Complémentaires. *Droit Social, 689*(5), 567–572.

Menard, J. (1996). Rapport de la Conférence Nationale de Santé—1996. *https:// www.vie-publique.fr/sites/default/files/rapport/pdf/974036500.pdf (last retrieved from 19 October 2020).*

Ministère des Solidarités et de la Santé, R. F. (2008). RAPPORT DE LA COMMISSION DE CONCERTATION SUR LES MISSIONS DE L'HÔPITAL, PRÉSIDÉE PAR M. GÉRARD LARCHER. *https://solidarites-sante.gouv.fr/IMG/pdf/rapport_Larcher_definitif.pdf (last retrieved from 16 October 2020).*

Mullard, A. (2011). Mediator Scandal Rocks French Medical Community. *The Lancet, 377*(9769), 890–892. https://doi.org/10.1016/S0140-6736(11)60334-6

Nouchi, F. (1995). Contrôler l'hôpital, mieux former les médecins. *Le Monde https://www.lemonde.fr/archives/article/1995/11/17/controler-l-hopital-mieux-former-les-medecins_3885927_1819218.html (last retrieved from 9 July 2020).*

Palier, B. (2008). *La Réforme des Systèmes de Santé.* Presses Universitaires de France.

Pierru, F., & Rolland, C. (2016). Bringing the Healthcare State Back in. Political Issues of Integration Through Merger: The Case of Regional Health Agencies. *Revue française de science politique (English Edition), 66*(3-4), 75–99. Retrieved from http://www.jstor.org/stable/90017580

Ract-Madoux, P., & Gauthey, G. (2018). La CADES, un acteur de la gestion et de l'amortissement de la dette sociale. *Regards, 54*(2), 45–54. https://doi.org/10.3917/regar.054.0045

République Française, L.-E.-F. (2018). Ma Santé 2022. Un Engagement Collectif. *https://solidarites-sante.gouv.fr/IMG/pdf/ma_sante_2022_synthese.pdf   (last retrieved from 31 December 2020).*

République Française, L.-E.-F. (2020). Légifrance. *https://www.legifrance.gouv.fr (last retrieved from 2 July 2020).*

Ritter, P. (2008). *RAPPORT SUR LA CREATION DES AGENCES REGIONALES DE SANTE (ARS).* https://solidarites-sante.gouv.fr/IMG/pdf/ARS_-_Rapport_Ritter-2.pdf (last retrieved from 3 July 2020)

Ruellan, R. (2015). La Gouvernance de la Sécurité Sociale à Partir du Plan Juppé de 1995. *Vie sociale, 10*(2), 153–171. https://doi.org/10.3917/vsoc.152.0153

Schrappe, M., François-Kettner, H., Gruhl, M., Knieps, F., Pfaff, H., & Glaeske, G. (2020). Thesenpapier 1.0 zur Pandemie durch SARS-CoV-2/Covid-19. Datenbasis verbessern—Prävention gezielt weiterentwickeln—Bürgerrechte wahren. *Monitor Versorgungsforschung, 13*(3), 53–63.

Secrétariat de la Conférence Nationale de Santé, M. r. d. T., de l'Emploi et de la Santé. (2010). Rapport d'Activité de la Conférence Nationale de Santé. *http://www.annuaire-secu.com/pdf/Rapport-CNS_mandature_2006-2010.pdf   (last retrieved from 19 October 2020).*

Seux, D. (1994). Réformes: la commission Minc appelle à « un nouveau compromis social ». *Les Echos https://www.lesechos.fr/1994/11/reformes-la-commission-minc-appelle-a-un-nouveau-compromis-social-892818 (last retrieved from 9 July 2020).*

Simonet, D. (2017). Recentralization and Vertical Alignment in the French Health-care System. *Journal of Public Affairs, 17*(4), e1640. https://doi.org/10.1002/pa.1640

Société Générale de Presse, L. (2020). Documentation Biographique des Quotidiens de la Société Générale de Presse. *https://www.lesbiographies.com (last retrieved from 7 October 2020).*

Soubie, R., Lagardère, M.-L., Meyer, C., Pibarot, M.-L., & Roger-Lacan, C. (1993). *Santé 2010. Groupe Prospective du Système de Santé présidé par Raymond Soubie.* Retrieved from Paris:

Soubie, R., Portos, J.-L., & Prieur, C. (1995). *Livre blanc sur le système de santé d'assurance-maladie.* Commisariat Général du Plan: La Documentation Française.

Touraine, M. (2014). Health Inequalities and France's National Health Strategy. *The Lancet, 383*(9923), 1101–1102. https://doi.org/10.1016/S0140-6736(14)60423-2

Tourmente, D. (2016). Les Groupements Hospitaliers de Territoires : Missions et Gouvernance des Nouveaux Outils de Coopération. *hal-01345525. https://hal.archives-ouvertes.fr/hal-01345525/document   (last   retrieved   from   31 December 2020).*

Treize membres. (1993). *Le Monde* *https://www.lemonde.fr/archives/article/1993/04/11/treize-membres_3921980_1819218.html (last retrieved from 9 July 2020).*

Weible, C. M., Nohrstedt, D., Cairney, P., Carter, D. P., Crow, D. A., Durnová, A. P., ... Stone, D. (2020). COVID-19 and the Policy Sciences: Initial Reactions and Perspectives. *Policy Sciences.* doi:https://doi.org/10.1007/s11077-020-09381-4

Wilcox, L. (2005). Metro, Info, Haro! Fierce Reactions to Regime Competition in the French Newspaper Industry. *Media, Culture & Society, 27*(3), 353–369. https://doi.org/10.1177/0163443705051748

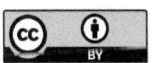

CHAPTER 6

Programmatic Action in German Health Policy

Analogous to the French case, the analysis of programmatic action in German health policy follows the PAF research protocol to trace the extent to which programmatic action is present. This is confirmed by existing publications (Bandelow & Hornung, 2020; Hornung & Bandelow, 2020), which are similar in their findings regarding the following elucidations. Nevertheless, the following subchapters serve to identify the programmatic group and its policy program both to validate the findings and to identify the core of the programmatic group to be identified for expert interviews. Most central to the analysis of programmatic action in Germany is the discovery of the institutional factors that enabled programmatic action despite the different system compared to France.

6.1   Policy Program in German Health Policy

Similar to France, health care reforms adopted in Germany pursued a strategy of centralization in order to concentrate competences and provide control over expenditures. In contrast to France, however, German health care reforms resorted to the introduction of elements of competition to achieve these goals (see Table 6.1). A first step in this direction was taken with the Health Care Structure Act (Gesundheitsstrukturgesetz, GSG) in 1992, which granted insured persons the free choice of sickness fund and established a risk structure compensation (Risikostrukturausgleich, RSA) between the different funds (Perschke-Hartmann, 1994, p. 265). Mätzke

© The Author(s) 2022   159
J. Hornung, *The Institutions of Programmatic Action*,
International Series on Public Policy,
https://doi.org/10.1007/978-3-031-05774-8_6

Table 6.1   Substantial health care reforms in Germany 1990–2010

Designation of reforms	Main reform content
Gesetz zur Sicherung und Strukturverbesserung der gesetzlichen Krankenversicherung (Gesundheitsstrukturgesetz), 21 December 1992	Introduction of performance-oriented remuneration instead of principle of cost coverage in hospitals, introduction of budgets to stationary and ambulatory care, reduction of the amount of licensed physicians, establishment of a whitelist (formulary) for reimbursable medicine, free choice of sickness fund for all insured people, introduction of a risk compensation scheme between sickness funds
Gesetz über die Neuordnung zentraler Einrichtungen des Gesundheitswesens (Gesundheitseinrichtungen-Neuordnungs-Gesetz—GNG), 24 June 1994	Restructures the Federal Health Agency, following a scandal of HIV-contaminated blood products
Gesetz zur Entlastung der Beiträge in der gesetzlichen Krankenversicherung (Beitragsentlastungsgesetz—BeitrEntlG) 1 November 1996	Fixes and reduces for the upcoming year 1997 the contribution rates, increases co-payments for drugs and medical products, shortening of services covered by SHI (eyewear and certain dental treatments) to reduce costs and contributions
Gesetz zur Stärkung der Finanzgrundlagen der gesetzlichen Krankenversicherung in den neuen Ländern (GKV-Finanzstärkungsgesetz—GKVFG), 24 March 1998	Breaks up the separation of sickness fund structures in former East and West Germany, joins the risk structure compensation scheme of both systems in the long term
Gesetz zur Reform der gesetzlichen Krankenversicherung ab dem Jahr 2000 (Gesundheitsreformgesetz 2000), 22 December 1999	Strengthening of the role of the general practitioner, strengthening of integrated care through facilitation of ambulatory care in hospitals, introducing the possibility of selective contracts between sickness funds and health care providers
Gesetz zur Anpassung der Regelungen über die Festsetzung von Festbeträgen für Arzneimittel in der gesetzlichen Krankenversicherung (Festbetrags-Anpassungsgesetz—FBAG), 27 July 2001	Pharmaceutical reference prices are adjusted by legislative decree of the health ministry, instead of by the sickness fund associations
Gesetz zur Reform des Risikostrukturausgleichs in der gesetzlichen Krankenversicherung, 10 December 2001	Introduction of a risk pool in the risk structure compensation scheme, risk structure compensation scheme will be expanded by a component taking into account the morbidity of insured people

(*continued*)

Table 6.1 (continued)

Designation of reforms	Main reform content
Gesetz zur Einführung des diagnose-orientierten Fallpauschalensystems für Krankenhäuser (Fallpauschalengesetz—FPG), 23 April 2002	Changes in the remuneration of hospitals, which now bases on performance-orientation in the form of diagnosis-related group payments, standardization
Gesetz zur Änderung der Vorschriften zum diagnose-orientierten Fallpauschalensystem für Krankenhäuser (Fallpauschalenänderungsgesetz—FPÄndG), 17 July 2003	Introduction and extension of transfer phase of the diagnosis-related group remuneration system, output quantity control, increased transparency, and quality assurance obligations of hospitals
Gesetz zur Modernisierung der gesetzlichen Krankenversicherung (GKV-Modernisierungsgesetz—GMG), 14 November 2003	Reform of the system of selective contracts (physicians may conclude such contracts with sickness funds without their respective association), fusions and mergers of Associations of Statutory Health Insurance Physicians, creation of IQWIG, creation of Joint Federal Committee, increase in co-payments in stationary and ambulatory care, strengthening of general-practitioner-centered care, introduction of an additional contribution for the insured
Gesetz zur Verbesserung der Wirtschaftlichkeit in der Arzneimittelversorgung, 26 April 2006	Bonus/malus regulation for physicians and their prescription practice of drugs, reduction of fixed prices for drugs
Gesetz zur Stärkung des Wettbewerbs in der gesetzlichen Krankenversicherung (GKV-Wettbewerbsstärkungsgesetz—GKV-WSG), 26 March 2007	Creation of SHI Peak Association, restructuring of the Joint Federal Committee, merging of sickness funds of different types, creation of health care fund, health ministry sets the universal contribution rate, sickness funds may charge an additional contribution from its insured people, introduction of morbidity into the risk structure compensation scheme, extension of selective contract system, extension of competences of Joint Federal Committee, compulsory insurance
Gesetz zur Weiterentwicklung der Organisationsstrukturen in der gesetzlichen Krankenversicherung (GKV-OrgWG), 15 December 2008	Sickness funds can become insolvent, short-term additional allocation of financial means from the Health Care Fund to sickness funds with above-average revenues and expenses

(continued)

Table 6.1 (continued)

Designation of reforms	Main reform content
Gesetz zum ordnungspolitischen Rahmen der Krankenhausfinanzierung ab dem Jahr 2009 (Krankenhausfinanzierungsreformgesetz—KHRG), 17 March 2009	Involvement of sickness funds in the financing of wage increases in hospitals, gradual alignment of the varying base rates to a uniform base rate corridor of DRG services
Gesetz zur Stabilisierung der Finanzlage der Sozialversicherungssysteme und zur Einführung eines Sonderprogramms mit Maßnahmen für Milchviehhalter sowie zur Änderung anderer Gesetze (Sozialversicherungs-Stabilisierungsgesetz—SozVersStabG), 14 April 2010	Increase in federal subsidy as a result of the financial crisis
Gesetz zur Neuordnung des Arzneimittelmarktes in der gesetzlichen Krankenversicherung (Arzneimittelmarktneuordnungsgesetz—AMNOG), 22 December 2010	Abolishment of bonus/malus regulation, strengthening of discount agreements by obliging pharmacists to deliver generic drugs if discount agreements require it, introduction of additional benefit assessment once new drugs enter the market (otherwise, the product falls under the fixed price regulation)

Source: Summaries of reforms are taken from the original legal documents and the overview by Reiners (2017a)

(2010, p. 135) sees this as a starting point for an increasing role and distinct organizational identity of the health ministry, based on policy-making in cross-partisan consensus and overcoming resistance from organized interest groups and a related shift from self-governance to hierarchical decision-making, for example, with the goal of cost containment. For the hospital sector, the reform included a change in financing that shifted from the remuneration of full cost cover to standardized prospective case financing (Busse & Schwartz, 1997).

Besides the content of the reform, the research literature on the GSG focuses on its genesis against the backdrop of the previous history of reform and Germany as a grand coalition state. According to this literature, the major structural reform and the "paradigm change" (Gerlinger, 2014, p. 35) it initiated resulted primarily from a cooperation of various party-political, but also administrative actors. In the final compromise concluded in Lahnstein, interest groups and representatives of sectoral actors were excluded (Reiners, 1993, pp. 29-33). This compromise was largely driven by the then health minister Horst Seehofer, and the chief negotiator of the Social Democratic Party (Sozialdemokratische Partei Deutschland, SPD), Rudolf Dreßler, and developed into a philosophy that they later adopted when communicating reform proposals (Seehofer et al., 1996). This exclusion of actors had been learned from earlier reform attempts under former minister Norbert Blüm, which failed due to strong resistance from interest representatives (Reiners, 2017b, pp. 24-25).

In the years following the GSG, many reform steps were taken toward reforming or adjusting the RSA scheme, which is one of the core elements of the competition-oriented regulation introduced to the German health care system (Busse, 2001, p. 175; Wysong & Abel, 1996, pp. 214-215). Others served more to contain costs, for example, by increasing co-payments and adjusting the SHI benefits catalogue (Kamke, 1998). Germany also introduced a general practitioner-centered model of health care (gatekeeper model) to allow sickness funds to use this as an element in competition with the other sickness funds and to reduce costs and contributions. The 1990s can also be seen as the starting point for breaking up established structures of contracting between sickness funds and physicians' associations, which were under the umbrella of collective contracts and opened up to the possibility of selective contracts (Mehl & Weiß, 2015, pp. 461-462).

The general trend toward more competition in the context of solidarity and equal access continued in the 2000s, for example, with the Health Care Reform Act (Gesundheitsreformgesetz, GRG) of 2000, which made it possible to conclude contracts for integrated care (Kifmann, 2017; Lisac et al., 2008, pp. 184-186). It also introduced a new system of financing inpatient care according to diagnosis-related groups (DRGs), through which inpatient care is no longer reimbursed as per the length of stay but with a fixed rate calculated for a specific diagnosis (Arnold, 2000). This system was inspired by the Australian system, as it was considered more transparent and equitable compared to other systems (Milstcin & Schreyögg, 2020, p. 28). Increased efficiency, transparency, and quality were cited as key goals of this reform (Braun et al., 2008).

In 2003, the SHI Modernization Act (GKV-Modernisierungsgesetz, GMG) again expanded the possibility of selective contracts between (individual or associations of) service providers and (individual or associations of) sickness funds (Bode, 2010, p. 66). In particular, the local sickness fund in the subnational state of Baden-Württemberg took advantage of the opportunities offered by these modes of governance (Hermann & Graf, 2012; Rohrer, 2017). As noted by Ulla Schmidt, then health minister, "the 2004 reform introduced explicit financial incentives for sickness funds and providers of health care jointly to develop contracts for proper disease and chronic care management, concepts that we Germans actually had picked up in the United States" (Cheng & Reinhardt, 2008, p. 206). This suggests that some of the ideas adopted in Germany were borrowed from other countries and inspired by the US system. To contain costs and allow competition between pharmaceutical companies and the sickness funds, the reform introduced the possibility of discount contracts to reduce spending on pharmaceutical products. These had been already discussed in Lahnstein and propagated by Rudolf Dreßler (Dietz, 2008).

The GMG also took some steps toward a more hierarchical form of institutional design. This relates above all to the establishment of the G-BA, the highest decision-making body of self-governance in the German health care system. It resulted from a merger of the previous negotiating bodies of the peak associations of service providers and payers, that is, physicians and hospitals, and the sickness funds. Similarly, the Institute for Quality and Efficiency in Health Care (Institut für Qualität und Wirtschaftlichkeit im Gesundheitswesen, IQWIG) was founded to provide evidence-based support for the decisions of the G-BA. At that time, the centralization tendencies of health care financing were further reinforced by the introduction of a tax-financed federal subsidy paid for non-insurance services (Jacobs, 2009, p. 28)

Continuing the strategy of cost containment through competition and centralization of decision-making, the Act to Strengthen Competition in the SHI (GKV-Wettbewerbsstärkungsgesetz, GKV-WSG) of 2007 is often mentioned in the same breath as the GMG and the GSG (Reiners, 2009). Among other things, this included the creation of the health care fund for the central administration of contributions and their distribution among the sickness funds according to the RSA scheme, as well as the installation of the GKV-SV. From an organizational and legal perspective, there has been much discussion about the legal and organizational status of sickness funds and physicians' associations as public corporations (Kruse & Kruse, 2006; Schillen & Kaiser, 2018). Furthermore, morbidity components have been added to the RSA scheme (Buchner et al., 2013) to remove incentives for sickness funds to select their insureds based on their health risks, thereby distorting the playing field for competition (Jahn et al., 2009, p. 45). Götze (2013) emphasizes that only then would the goals of the GSG and true price competition have been achieved. To strengthen the solidarity aspect, the GKV-WSG made health insurance mandatory and universal through, which was also partly inspired by policies in the Netherlands (Manouguian et al., 2006). Key points of the GKV-WSG had also been prepared by another commission, the 16-member cross-coalition federal-state working group that drafted the key points of a health care reform (Grimmeisen & Wendt, 2010, p. 164). It included high-ranking politicians from the federal and state levels, including Josef Hecken (then still minister in Saarland), as well as administrative staff (Sucker-Sket, 2006).

A final step in the reviewed reforms can be seen in the AMNOG of 2011, which came close to adding a fourth hurdle for pharmaceutical products to enter the market. Newly produced drugs must now be assessed for an additional benefit compared to existing pharmaceutical products, and only if this is established may the company enter into price negotiations with the GKV-SV. Otherwise, the drugs are transferred to the reference price system. However, it is questionable what impact this regulation will have on the access to pharmaceuticals for the insured (Henschke et al., 2013).

The course of German health care reforms has been analyzed in detail by several authors and studies. A high level of agreement concerns the observation that the German health care system has become increasingly economized and marketized (Ewert, 2009). Reforms since 1990 are often described as following a "third way" vision, which essentially means the introduction of elements of competition into an otherwise publicly structured, hierarchical governance structure (Allen & Riemer Hommel, 2006; Kuhlmann et al., 2009, p. 515). In this context, health policy reforms required political trade-offs between the goals of solidarity on the one hand and financeability and competition on the other (Stock et al., 2007). Another key finding of health policy analyses is the increased role of the state and hierarchical modes of governance to weaken self-regulation (Rothgang et al., 2010), although this view is contested. Some see the reforms more as strengthening corporatist bodies (Altenstetter & Busse, 2005). In general, scholars agree that the aforementioned reforms are an ongoing reform program, whose reforms are interrelated in terms of problem identification, goals, and instruments (Gerlinger, 2010; Lisac et al., 2010). Hartmann (2003) classifies the policies of the 1990s after the GSG as a distinct phase compared to the phase of cost containment before it, and the health care policies of the governing coalition of the SPD and the Greens (Bündnis 90/Die Grünen) until its end in 2002 as a continuation of this phase (Hartmann, 2003, p. 270).

The ideas of these reforms can be traced back even further to the Enquete Commission Structural Reform of the SHI (Strukturreform der gesetzlichen Krankenversicherung) (Götze, 2016, p. 186), which in its final report already advocated the introduction of competitive elements in the health care system, such as a risk compensation scheme and the elimination of strict differences between sickness funds according to the occupational group they insure (Deutscher Bundestag, 1990). Manow (1994, p. 97) notes that this can be seen as a cross-party and cross-ideological consensus. Based on the Enquete Commission and, to some extent, the Structural Commission at the DGB Federal Executive Board on "The Future of Solidary Health Security", which is still cited in some works by proponents of these ideas (Rosenbrock, 1992), it can be assumed that the reforms implemented in subsequent years made use of the ideas agreed upon by these groups of people in these commissions. Other authors who see a substantial connection between the reforms as part of a larger policy program were themselves part of the group that drove these reforms (Knieps, 2016). They also trace the ideas behind the reforms to the development of a scientific discipline, namely health economics under professor Philipp Herder-Dorneich (Rebscher, 2016, p. 47).

Some of the reforms, such as the introduction of the Health Care Fund, are seen by scholars as a compromise in the ideological conflict between the advocates of solidarity (with the party-political representative of the SPD) versus the advocates of self-responsibility and financeability (with the party-political representative of the Christian Democratic Union (Christlich Demokratische Union Deutschlands, CDU) and the Christian Social Union (Christlich-Soziale Union, CSU). It is interesting, however, that even reforms formally initiated by the red-green government explicitly refer to the principle of self-responsibility in their presentation of the reform (Deutscher Bundestag, 1999). Indeed, this could be an indication of the occurrence of a "Nixon-goes-to-China effect" (Wenzelburger et al., 2018). However, the clear reference by Ulla Schmidt to "solidarity and affordability of a high-quality health care system [as] the twin goals of our reform" (Cheng & Reinhardt, 2008, p. 205) and Horst Seehofer ("For me, solidarity and personal responsibility are brother and sister" (Seehofer, 1996)) shows that there was a broad cross-party consensus, a programmatic identity, guiding the statements of central actors in health policy. Nevertheless, such an effect is also visible in the health care reforms in Germany (Knieps, 2016, p. 29).

As in the French case, some structural policies cannot be linked to reform programs and seem to be empirical examples of theoretical perspectives that focus on scandals and external events or beliefs and interests. These include the abolition of the Federal Health Office, which was absorbed in several other agencies following the concealment of contaminated blood products (Laschet, 2019). Toward the end of the 1990s, the two Acts on the Reorganization of the SHI, which linked co-payments to contribution rates and reduced the benefits catalogue, were met with alienation by all those who had supported the reform path taken earlier. Several actors criticized the reforms (Cassel et al., 1997; Hermann, 1997) and they were reversed by the new governing coalition after the change of government in 1998 (Knieps, 2016, p. 27). After the change of government, the Solidarity Strengthening Act is only a counter-reaction to the Reorganization Acts. While the 2000 health reform contains rudiments of further programmatic action (see below), the development of health policy up to the GMG is characterized by being primarily the result of a proliferation of individual interests and also the result of partisan effects.

6.2   PROGRAMMATIC ACTORS IN GERMAN HEALTH POLICY

In order to gain further insight into the group of actors who advocated increased economization of the health care system and the ideas of increased centralized regulation to ensure solidarity within these competitive structures, the analysis of newspaper articles represents the second step of the German study. Analogous to the French case, the daily newspaper with the highest circulation in Germany, the *Süddeutsche Zeitung*, is taken as the reference point. As this German newspaper is also considered center-left in its orientation, this selection rules out a potential bias when comparing discourse networks of France and Germany stemming from different orientations of the two newspapers under study. Like in France, it may be that some topics or actors gain more attention from leftist newspapers compared to right-wing-oriented newspapers. Given that the research interest pursued here lies in the reconstruction of the reform trajectories and their supporting actors, the way that newspapers frame political events and reforms has little to no effect on the results. Also, an overestimated or underestimated role of policy ideas and/or actors would become visible when cross-checking the results of the discourse analysis with interview data and document analyses.

To ensure comparability of results, the search bases on the same keywords, namely "social security/health insurance" (Krankenversicherung) and "health policy" (Gesundheitspolitik). In the period between 1 January 1990 and 31 December 2010, 409 articles containing these keywords were published. Focusing only on those that discuss reforms more concretely, 146 articles remain in the sample to be analyzed with the Discourse Network Analyzer.

As in the French case, the detailed history of newspaper articles on health policy reforms in Germany also allows for tracing the dominant debates at the time of discussion. It also allows a step-by-step review of the reform history. The health policy coverage of the 1990s begins in 1992 with a public discussion of the attempts and questionable success of the governing coalition to contain health spending and the measures used to achieve this goal. The SPD accused the governing coalition of being unable to reduce health care costs, while public debates centered on whether increasing co-payments, reducing the benefits catalogue, reforming remunerations, and budgeting were appropriate tools to address this problem. At that time, the then minister of health, Horst Seehofer of the CSU, invited Rudolf Dreßler, then the SPD's main health policy expert, to work together on a health care reform.

Following the 1992 reform, the SVR-G's "Gesundheitsweisen" (health experts) presented another starting point for further health care reforms in a scientific report in 1995 (SVR, 1995). It explicitly advocated more competition in the health care system. While the SVR-G held back with clear recommendations and opinions, a tendency toward required competition between sickness funds was already apparent here, allowing individual premium reductions through optional services (5 February 1994). Seehofer emphasized that the ideas of the sectoral actors should first be clarified before concrete reform steps were taken in the next direction.

The media reported at that time that various actors were calling for the implementation of the so-called third stage of health reform. This meant linking an increase in contribution rates with increases in co-payments, parity-based financing of contributions, and the targeted expansion of prevention and rehabilitation in the sense of solidarity-based health care. In an interview on 6 July 1996, however, Seehofer made it clear that he believed prevention was best left to the individual and not to the sickness funds. As a result, preventive services and precautionary measures in particular were removed from the benefits catalogue, which met with strong resentment and criticism from the SPD. However, he was unable to push through the division of health insurance benefits into compulsory and optional benefits. When Horst Seehofer presented the draft bill for the planned reform of health insurance in February 1996, the SPD under Rudolf Dreßler presented a counter-draft with the threat of using the newly won majority in the Bundesrat as veto power. The draft reforms for "further development" ultimately failed. This was also due to three state election results in March 1996, which strengthened the Liberal Democratic Party (Freie Demokratische Partei, FDP) and weakened the SPD, thus preventing a repetition of the grand-coalitionary compromise as in Lahnstein.

Horst Seehofer's term in office was followed by Andrea Fischer as health minister of the Greens under Gerhard Schröder's red-green coalition. With her planned health reform included the introduction of global budgets, a positive list, responsibility for hospital investments resting with the sickness funds, and the review and process evaluation of new medical devices. The latter also led to an intensive discussion about whether medical progress necessarily entails an increase in costs or whether it can also reduce costs (Steinkohl, 1999). The conflict also became apparent again within the governing coalition, partly due to Rudolf Dreßler's still strong position. But the CDU also threatened to reject the reform in the Bundesrat. Interestingly, there were also talks between old friends Rudolf Dreßler and Horst Seehofer at this time. Finally, the reform ended up in the mediation committee. As expected, no compromise was reached, so Andrea Fischer subsequently passed a version of the reform reduced by the points requiring approval. This contained only the budgets for drugs, physician fees, and clinics, as well as a strengthening of the selective contracts. The example of Rudolf Dreßler and Horst Seehofer during the time of incumbent health minister Andrea Fischer shows that old friendships and biographical intersections have a lasting effect, because both "overthrew" a health minister who was not part of the group, although there was definitely consensus on some points such as contracts between sectoral actors, co-payments, competition, hospital restructuring, and individual responsibility for certain benefits.

Even if the compromise between Horst Seehofer and Rudolf Dreßler was a political one, the Enquete Commission at least had a personnel effect, that is, many of the members of the Enquete Commission were at least involved in the public discourse, if not in the solutions agreed upon in Lahnstein. If we look at the discourse network in Fig. 6.1, which shows that the media discourse in the selected newspaper between 1990 and 2000, some names emerge that were members of the Enquete Commission. In addition to Horst Seehofer, these are Paul Hoffacker and Dieter Thomae. With them, however, the network remains politicized. The politicization can easily be explained by the chosen media organ and the logic with which journalistic reports are written. As mentioned above, sectoral actors and potentially programmatic actors are hardly observable in public discourse, but operate in the background. The discourse network is thus more indicative of the policy program, whose ideational roots are still to be found in the biographies of actors. If the policy program is shared broadly publicly across party-political actors, there is high probability that a programmatic group is working behind the scenes that has reached a cross-party consensus on a far-reaching reform program.

In 2001, Andrea Fischer was finally replaced by Ulla Schmidt as health minister. However, the problem of rising costs had still not been solved, and the question of contribution rate stability and which services should be paid for by the sickness funds and on what basis remained under discussion. In this situation, Ulla Schmidt proposed a reform of RSA with an extension to include a morbidity orientation and introduced flat rates per case, which had already been discussed in the 1990s as a means of increasing efficiency, as a remuneration system in hospitals. At the same time, she abolished measures pushed through by Andrea Fischer, such as the drug budget. Although these measures met with criticism from the sectoral partners, there was no political resistance even in the absence of conspicuous health policy personalities. This was also due to internal disagreement within the CDU/CSU; the separation of elective and compulsory benefits was welcomed by the CDU but rejected by the CSU. In 2002, a group of scientists close to the SPD presented a draft for the health policy of the future (4 April 2002—key elements of a new health policy). This group included well-known names who had also played a role in the Enquete Commission or in other health science contexts, including Gerd Glaeske, Jürgen Wasem, Christopher Hermann, and Karl Lauterbach. They called for greater consideration of evidence-based and independent institutions in quality assurance, a strengthening of integrated care, improved use of the general practitioner-centered model, and a greater role for disease management programs (DMPs). Fittingly, since the 2000s there has also been increasing talk of quality competition instead of price competition, that is, the possibility of choosing between different health insurance plans according to the quality of care (such as general practitioner-centered models, selective contracts, and DMPs). Related to this, the GMG in the early 2000s introduced bonus programs for sickness funds, which were also intended to further develop competition among them. To contain costs on the revenue and expenditure side, the reform also decoupled dentures from the SHI benefits catalogue and increased co-payments for medicines. A practice fee required every patient to pay €10 quarterly when visiting a doctor.

In 2003, the Herzog Commission drew up important proposals for reforming social security. These later served as the basis for the CDU program, which envisaged a fundamental change in the financing basis of SHI from financing via income-dependent contributions to income-independent capitation payments. However, the CSU rejected the proposals presented, except for the point about freezing the employer contributions. At the same time, the Rürup Commission set up by the federal government was also working on social policy proposals, whose members tended to be close to the SPD. Interestingly, the Rürup Commission also came up with the proposal of a capitation payment. This was also the strategy proposed by the SVR-G, of which Bert Rürup was a member at the time. The commissions' findings had a decisive influence on the election campaign and the subsequent coalition negotiations in 2005.

Following the commissions' findings, internal conflicts arose between supporters and opponents of the proposals developed. CSU party leader Edmund Stoiber spoke out in favor of the capitation fee, while CSU Health Minister Horst Seehofer rejected it. Within the CDU/CSU parliamentary group, a compromise solution crystallized for a health premium as a reaction to the conflicts, which would place a greater burden on higher earners and thus also include an income-related component. This was supported by the CSU and parts of the CDU. Edmund Stoiber's compromise proposal set the flat rate to be paid at 109 euros, but no more than 7% of income.

In the coalition negotiations for the grand coalition in 2005, however, the parties agreed on a compromise, namely the establishment of the health care fund through the GKV-WSG. Here, health insurance contributions were combined uniformly and then redistributed among the sickness funds according to their expenditures and the morbidity-oriented risk structure compensation (Morbiditätsorientierter Risikostrukturausgleich, Morbi-RSA). The federal subsidy already introduced in the GMG to finance non-insurance benefits was actually to be abolished, but was reintroduced in response to the "solidarity-based" tax financing of the capitation fee demanded by the CDU and CSU. The GKV-WSG 2007 also set the contribution rate to the sickness funds at a uniform percentage. In order to maintain competitive structures, though, the sickness funds were allowed to levy an additional contribution on an individual basis. These structures largely still apply today, even though the additional contribution was made income-dependent in 2015 (Simon, 2016).

Toward the end of the 2000s, the reform discourse changed slightly as other problems came onto the agenda. Medical deserts and the insufficient provision of health care in more sparsely populated areas posed substantial challenges to health policy actors, as did a financing reform of long-term care insurance. The goal of cost containment also remained on the agenda, but it was achieved through two developments: First, the unpopular health minister Philipp Rösler failed to push through the capitation fee against the resistance of the coalition partner CDU/CSU, even though it had been stipulated in the coalition agreement. Instead, the CDU/CSU advocated a reform of the health care fund. This was demanded in particular by the CSU, in persona Markus Söder and Horst Seehofer. The latter in particular vehemently opposed the introduction of capitation fees, also to the displeasure of the coalition partners CDU and FDP. A final compromise led to a hierarchical definition of an average additional contribution, which was offset by a reduction in the overall contribution if a certain fixed amount was exceeded. In the same breath, the additional contributions were decoupled from employers' expenditures. On the other hand, the reaction to the financial crisis prompted health policy-makers to increase the contribution rate by 0.6 percentage points to 15.7%. Only later did it become apparent that this adjustment of the contribution rate was in fact an overreaction of German health policy to the financial crisis (Blum & Kuhlmann, 2016).

In contrast to the discourse network shown in Fig. 6.1, the discourse network of health policy in Germany between 2000 and 2010 (Fig. 6.2) shows a different picture in terms of density and number of connected nodes. It is populated by more actors, and among these actors are not only politicians but increasingly also actors from the self-governing institutions of the sickness funds. These include, for example, Christopher Hermann from the local sickness fund of Baden-Württemberg, and academics who advocate competition in the health care system, including Jürgen Wasem and Gerd Glaeske. Besides, some core topics of the discourse are highlighted. The dispute between CDU, CSU, and SPD over the future

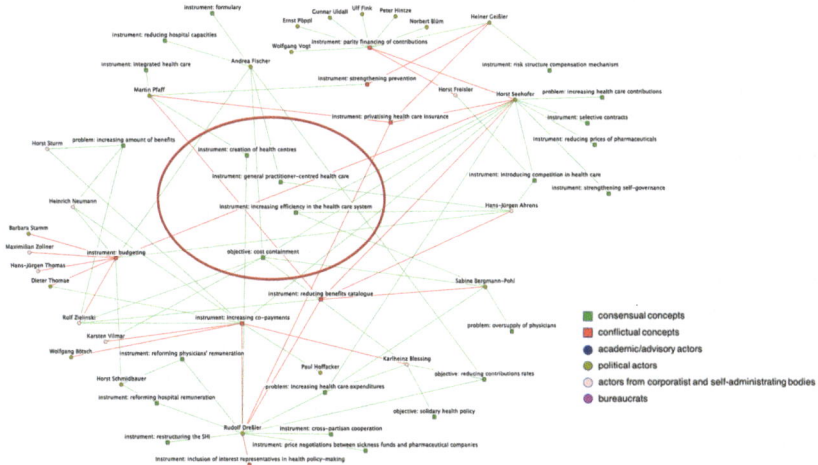

Fig. 6.1 Discourse network of health policy in Germany, 1990–2000. Source: Own illustration, created with the software visone (Brandes & Wagner, 2019). The red outlines emphasize the programmatic content of the discourse

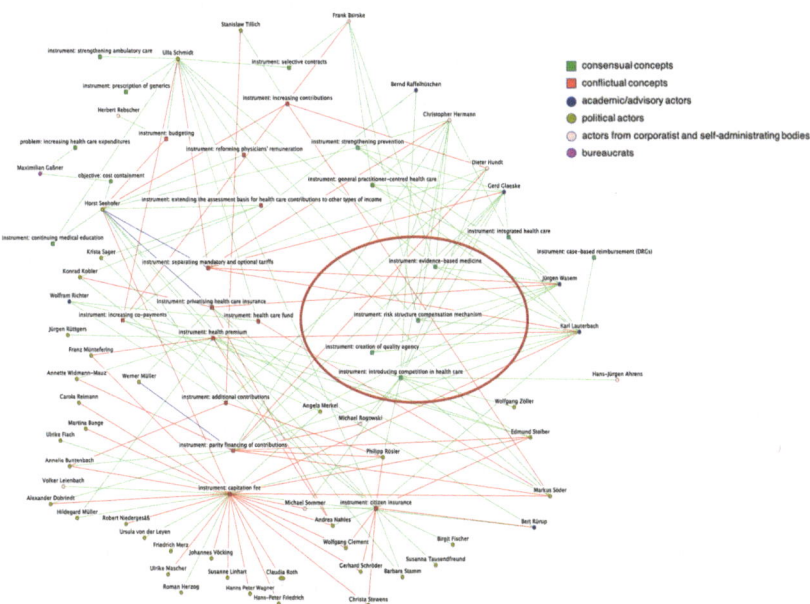

Fig. 6.2 Discourse network of health policy in Germany, 2000–2010. Source: Own illustration, created with the software visone (Brandes & Wagner, 2019). The red outlines emphasize the programmatic content of the discourse

financing of the SHI system with the main instruments of citizens' insurance, capitation fees, and health premiums, which is being driven throughout the debate, is also visible in the discourse network. In addition, evidence-based medicine, general practitioner-centered care, and the call for the creation of an agency to monitor quality in health care, partly with reference to the National Institute for Health and Care Excellence (NICE) in the UK, were among the policy instruments promoted by non-political actors. There is also agreement on these themes, suggesting that they fit the public narrative and perceived health care reform needs and solutions. As a consequence, the discourse network shows that less polarization of a discourse is associated with it being shared by a larger number of people. The respective instruments that constitute a policy program are discussed unanimously in the media and hardly criticized.

The discourse network analysis of German health policy between 1990 and 2010 has shown that there has been a lively debate about adequate reform strategies in response to the challenge of rising health care costs. In the first ten years, the discourse was largely dominated by political actors. Although the ideas discussed in the Enquete Commission—including selective contracts, the RSA scheme, and other competitive elements— were slow to enter the debate, the main instruments discussed were simple ones that were known to have a reducing effect on health care spending. As a result, policy-makers struggled mainly to reduce the benefits catalogue, introduce budgets for health care, or increase co-payments. It was not until the 2000s that the instruments of the policy program "competition in a solidaristic framework" (Knieps, 2017, p. 12) came into the spotlight and manifested themselves in the public debate. This is the time when one can speak even more of programmatic action, as the public discourse networks become denser and populated by diverse actors from academia and self-governance.

6.3   BIOGRAPHIES AND IDENTITIES OF GERMAN PROGRAMMATIC ACTORS

Continuing with the actors in the discourse network, it is noticeable that, in contrast to France, not so many administrative actors were visible in the network. Instead, the discourse was largely shaped by party-political experts and experts who, in one way or the other, found their way into self-governance. In addition, those who occupied the positions relevant to the adoption of reforms, most notably the leaders in the relevant departments in the health ministry, stayed in the background.

Based on the relevant formal positions in the German health care system shown in Fig. 4.2, it is possible to identify in retrospect the central actors who held these positions during the period under review from 1990 to 2010. In particular, it can also be shown whether new institutions were created that were occupied by biographically related actors and after their joint promotion of a policy program. The positions formally considered relevant are found at the highest levels of self-government. In addition to the department of health insurance in the health ministry, these are primarily positions in the represented organizations of today's Joint Federal Committee, that is, the KBV, the DKG, and the GKV-SV. In addition, the SVR-G, which is based in the health ministry, potentially plays a decisive role.

Looking at these positions, the key position in the health ministry—and comparable to France—has been occupied by a programmatic actor even after the first reform steps had been implemented. The German counterpart to Dominique Libault is Franz Knieps, who occupied the post between 2003 and 2009 and was thus responsible for two to three of the four most important health care reforms. A more detailed look at the formal key positions in the German health care system and the individuals who occupied these positions during the period under study is presented in Table 6.2 as the starting point of the analysis. It highlights the role of Franz Knieps in the health ministry during an important period of reform. At the same time, it shows that the centralization of health care institutions in turn the actors who now occupy central positions to be traced back to the institutions that were relevant before the institutional change initiated by the programmatic group.

The board of directors of the GKV-SV, founded in 2007, was chaired by Doris Pfeiffer, Johann-Magnus von Stackelberg, and Volker Hansen, whose biographies had in common that they had held top positions in the federal association of local sickness funds (AOK-Bundesverband, AOK-BV) before the 1990s. Interestingly, the first impartial chairmen at the top of the G-BA, Rainer Hess, also came from this network. He stayed until 2012, marking the end of programmatic action with the AMNOG as the final reform step.

Another interesting body that had evolved over the years was the SVR-G. Originally convened for the concerted action in the health sector, it became an important stop in the careers of programmatic actors and a place of intellectual debate that was inspirational for the further development of the policy program. Many of the former members of the SVR-G

Table 6.2 Occupied positions in key institutions of German health policy

Name	Time	Position
Head of Department of Health Care in the Federal Ministry of Health (until 1991 part of the Federal Ministry of Labour)		
Karl Jung	1982–1994	Director
Gerhard Schulte	1994–1996	Director
Manfred Zipperer	1996–1998	Director
Hermann Schulte-Sasse	1998–2001	Director
Edwin Smiegelski	2001–2003	Director
Franz Knieps	2003–2009	Director
Ulrich Orlowski	2009–2019	Director
GKV-SV (GKV-Spitzenverband / SHI Peak Association) (founded in 2007)		
Doris Pfeiffer	Since 2007	Board of Directors
Johann-Magnus von Stackelberg	2007–2019	Board of Directors
Volker Hansen	2007–2019	Board of Directors
Joint Federal Committee (founded in 2004)		
Rainer Hess	2004–2012	Impartial Chairman
Josef Hecken	Since 2012	Impartial Chairman
SVR-G (Sachverständigenrat zur Begutachtung der Entwicklung im Gesundheitswesen/Council of Experts for the Assessment of Developments in the Health Care System)		
Martin-Michael Arnold	1988–1992	Chairman
Klaus-Dirk Henke	1992–1998	Chairman
Friedrich-Wilhelm Schwartz	1998–2002	Chairman
Eberhard Wille	2002–2012	Chairman
Ferdinand Gerlach	Since 2012	Chairman

Source: Own illustration, based on requested organigrams of the health ministry, and the respective websites of the individuals

were present in the media, such as Karl Lauterbach, who continues to play an important role in health policy in the recent era of the COVID-19 pandemic and is frequently quoted in public discourses (Dyer, 2020). Others, such as Rolf Rosenbrock and Günter Neubauer, were previously part of the Enquete Commission and were able to transfer these ideas and institutionalize them in the SVR-G. Similarly, it was the SVR-G that carried some reform ideas, such as the reorganization of sickness funds, to the Enquete Commission. As can be seen from the commission's final report, Martin Pfaff and Gerd Glaeske, then members of the SVR-G, had advised the members of the Enquete Commission on this topic (Deutscher Bundestag, 1990, p. 17f). Looking at these examples, it can be stated that there was an intensive cross-commission exchange with biographically connected individuals who pursued a common policy program.

Despite the fact that there were biographical intersections between health policy actors in Germany that laid the foundation for programmatic action, the clear link to institutions and the discourse network is less visible compared to France. This is mainly because the programmatic group was less formally visible and acted more informally. This is not to say that the Enquete Commission was an informal occasion alone. Nevertheless, it is striking that much of the collaboration appears to have taken place behind the scenes. This is evident not least from the lower visibility of programmatic actors in the discourse network. Instead of being present in the daily newspapers, the programmatic group used the channels of the sectoral publication organs to disseminate their ideas. The programmatic actors participated in a number of joint publication projects. One of the most recent major ones is a written account of the program "solidarity-based competitive order" (Cassel et al., 2014). Published in 2014, when the introduction of competitive elements in the health care system had already been largely realized, the authors identify challenges to further implementation of this program, one of which appears to be the lack of consideration of these ideas in the coalition agreements (Jacobs & Rebscher, 2014, p. 67). The programmatic group was also active in some sector-specific forums that provided ongoing intellectual reflection behind the scenes of the public debate. One example is the Federal Managed Care Association (Bundesverband Managed Care, BMC), whose board still consists of former programmatic actors who continue to publish their programmatic ideas (Amelung et al., 2017), and whose chairman himself pushed for market-based reforms in health care, inspired by the US experience (Brown & Amelung, 1999).

Looking at the actors who occupied the relevant positions in the central institutions of the German health care system dentified in Fig. 4.2 between 1990 and 2010, the analysis shows the intersecting biographies of key actors whose start of cooperation dates back to the Enquete Commission and the compromise agreed in Lahnstein. One key person who develops here is Franz Knieps, head of the department of health care, statutory health insurance, long-term care insurance in the health ministry from 2003 to 2007, after having made his career in one of the largest sickness fund associations. Christopher Hermann also was part of the secretariat, at that time seconded from the scientific service of the German Bundestag. Christopher Hermann then became a research associate at the Ministry of Social Affairs and Health of North Rhine-Westphalia, succeeding Hartmut Reiners, who held a central position in the health ministry of the state of Brandenburg. Hartmut Reiners confirmed in an email that he was in charge of coordinating the health policies of the SPD-led states and therefore worked very closely with Christopher Hermann. These three individuals can be considered part of the core programmatic group around health policy reforms in Germany from the 1990s onward.

The analysis of actors' biographies also points to other intersections that are of interest for the study of the adopted reforms. In contrast to the ENA in France, the importance of higher education in Germany depends less on the institution or location (as may be the case in the UK and the US) than on the subject. In the 1990s, health economics became an important source of influence for ideas on the organization of health care. Thus, the focus on competition in health care is not accidental. As indicated in the document analysis, Philipp Herder-Dorneich's students, as one of the first two German health economists, substantially shaped the ideas and paths of the policy program. Jürgen Wasem, one of his students, can be considered a scientific part of the programmatic group, as his work on the Morbi-RSA scheme was transferred to policy (Jahn et al., 2009; Wasem, 1993; Wasem et al., 2016). Together with Eberhard Wille, Jürgen Wasem was a member of the Scientific Advisory Board on the Further Development of the Risk Structure Compensation Scheme (Wissenschaftlicher Beirat zur Weiterentwicklung des Risikostrukturausgleichs) (BAS, 2020). Participation in this scientific advisory board and in the SVR-G also enabled cross-institutional collaboration and further elaboration of the policy program with proposals for its redesign.

A special biographical connection seems to be the AOK-BV. Franz Knieps began his career there, as did many others. Hartmut Reiners writes in a private email: "*What we had in common was that we, as economists, social scientists or lawyers, were involuntary pioneers, because health care and especially SHI was a 'terra incognita' in the academic field until the 1980s. At the same time, the academisation of the health insurance associations was pursued, especially in the AOK, driven by its board and WIdO founder Alfred Schmidt (DGB). At that time there were only two professors of economics, [Philipp] Herder-Dorneich in Cologne and Theo Thiemeyer in Bochum, and a lawyer ([Bernd] von Maydell), who had their main focus of work here. Their staff and doctoral students then made a career in the ministerial and health insurance bureaucracy and formed an informal network that had and still has a forum in the journal 'Gesundheits- und Sozialpolitik' (Health and Social Policy), which was co-edited by Franz Knieps*". Hartmut Reiners' quote refers to a common source of ideas and contacts in the network decisively built up by the local sickness funds (AOK) and their federal association at the federal level. The publications by the WiDO (Scientific Institute of the Local Sickness Funds; Wissenschaftliches Institut der Allgemeinen Ortskrankenkassen) obviously influenced or at least accompanied the health care reforms (Cassel et al., 2008).

Based on the findings generated in the previous sections, especially the discourse network, document analysis and formal position analysis, the analysis of biographical intersections draws on actors who were visible at several points in this empirical study. Specifically, the actors selected as anchoring examples to substantiate the existence of a programmatic group held different positions in the ministry (Franz Knieps), in the self-governance (Christopher Hermann), at the Länder level (Hartmut Reiners), and in academia (Jürgen Wasem). They got to know each other through the Enquete Commission and the subsequent Lahnstein compromise. In addition, their cooperation was intensified through working groups, for example, the respective key point discussions on the health care reforms of 2003 and 2007 (Schwartz & Mosebach, 2003; Wasem, 2009). The call for more competition in health care was even shared even by normally opposing actors, such as employee and employer representatives (DGB, 2003). Sources for the biographical information on the following anchoring examples are the BKK DV (2020), Wolfangel (2020), the Universität Duisburg-Essen (2020), and personal interviews.

Anchoring Example: Christopher Hermann
- *Until 1987* Law, policy, and history student
- *1987–1990* Scientific service of the German Bundestag
- *1990–1997* Research assistant at the Ministry of Social Affairs and Health of North Rhine-Westphalia
- *1997–2000* Group leader at the Ministry of Social Affairs and Health of North Rhine-Westphalia
- *2000–2011* Member of the board of the AOK Baden-Württemberg
- *2011–2019* Chairman of the AOK Baden-Württemberg

Anchoring Example: Franz Knieps
- *1975–1981* Law student at the universities of Bonn and Freiburg
- *1982–1986* Research assistant to Bernd von Maydell at the Institute for Labour Law and Social Security Law at the University of Bonn
- *1986–1987* Consultant for basic legal policy issues at the AOK Federal Association

- *1987–1988* Secondment to the Federal Ministry of Labor and Social Affairs to support Minister Norbert Blüm's work on health reform
- *1989–1998* Head of the Policy Department of the AOK Federal Association
- *1998–2003* Managing Director Politics at the AOK Federal Association
- *2003–2009* Head of the Department of Health Care, Statutory Health Insurance, Long-Term Care Insurance in the Federal Ministry of Health
- *2009–2013* Management consultancy Wiese-Consult
- *2013* WMP HealthCare GmbH
- *Since July 2013* Chairman of the BKK federal association

Anchoring Example: Hartmut Reiners
- *Until 1988* Scientific institute of the local health insurance funds
- *1987–1990* Enquete Commission "Structural Reform of the Statutory Health Insurance"
- *1988–1992* Health ministry, North-Rhine Westphalia
- *1992–pension* Head of the policy unit of the health ministry in Brandenburg

Anchoring Example: Jürgen Wasem
- *1978–1983* Study of Economics Political Science, and Social Policy
- *1983–1985* Research Assistant and Doctorate at the University of Cologne, chair of Philipp Herder-Dorneich
- *1985–1989* Consultant in the Department of Health Care and Health Insurance in the Federal Ministry of Labor and Social Affairs
- *2003* Member of the Herzog Commission and advisor to Ulla Schmidt

It is striking that the local sickness fund associations and their scientific institute represent the roots of several programmatic actors that were brought together in the Enquete Commission. Moreover, the Enquete Commission, the Lahnstein Compromise, and the SVR-G represent biographical intersections shared by many programmatic actors. Thus, it can be concluded that these biographical commonalities are the source of programmatic action.

6.4   THE DECLINE OF THE PROGRAMMATIC GROUP IN GERMAN HEALTH POLICY

The previous chapters have provided evidence and empirical trajectories of instances of programmatic action in French and German health policy from 2011 to 2020. To assess the influence of institutional settings on the presence and absence of programmatic action, this subchapter presents a case in which programmatic action did not occur and investigates the reasons why this is the case. It also outlines how the PAF can be falsified. With respect to the French case, PAF scholars concluded that the old programmatic group is still active and relevant even in the recent COVID-19 pandemic (Hassenteufel, 2020). It is therefore useful to look more closely at the period after programmatic action in German health policy to evaluate which of the explanatory factors for programmatic action have changed to explain the absence of programmatic action since then. Against the backdrop of the formulated hypotheses on the influence of political institutions on programmatic action, the results later show under which institutions programmatic action occurs.

As in the previous empirical studies, the analysis of the German health care reform period from 2010 to 2020 starts with an overview of adopted policies with the aim of identifying a possible reform program. As Table 6.3 shows, however, the directions of the individual policies are not visibly linked. Under health minister Hermann Gröhe, health policy focused only on prevention and innovation. By overreacting to the financial crisis in 2010, the German health care system had overcome its financial problems. Money was abundant and was used to address the problems that arose. For example, financial incentives were used to attract more physicians to sparsely populated areas and to offer new services for those in need of care and the seriously ill. Only the rapid pace of reform under Jens Spahn as a health minister and his restructuring of the health ministry, including the designation of a unit for digitalization and the placement of one of his party trustees at the top, might give a hint of a hidden reform program of digitalization.

The major structural reforms under Jens Spahn can be illustrated very well by a few, also known as "omnibus laws" because of their comprehensive nature. Only these are listed in Table 6.3. In terms of content, the reforms essentially encompassed four central aspects, which can be summarized under the headings of patient-centeredness, care policy, digitalization, and increased state oversight. With regard to patient-centeredness,

Table 6.3   Substantial health care reforms in Germany 2010–2020

Reform	Main reform content
Erstes Gesetz zur Stärkung der pflegerischen Versorgung und zur Änderung weiterer Vorschriften (Erstes Pflegestärkungsgesetz—PSG I), 19 December 2014	Increases benefit amounts of the nursing insurance, expands short-term and preventative care services, extends entitlement to low-threshold care services in outpatient care, increase in funds for conversion measures to up to 4000 euros per measure
Gesetz zur Stärkung der Versorgung in der gesetzlichen Krankenversicherung (GKV-Versorgungsstärkungsgesetz—GKV-VSG), 22 July 2015	Creates financial incentives and improved working conditions in rural areas to make the profession of rural doctor more attractive, establishment of a Structural Fund, facilitating possibilities for establishing medical care centers
Zweites Gesetz zur Stärkung der pflegerischen Versorgung und zur Änderung weiterer Vorschriften (Zweites Pflegestärkungsgesetz—PSG II), 1 January 2016	Equal access to long-term care insurance benefits, new assessment tool to assess the individual care and living situation of people who have applied for long-term care insurance benefits, personnel assessment in inpatient facilities: By 2020, the self-government must develop and test a scientifically based procedure for the uniform assessment of personnel requirements in care facilities, further development of quality assurance regulations
Drittes Gesetz zur Stärkung der pflegerischen Versorgung und zur Änderung weiterer Vorschriften (Drittes Pflegestärkungsgesetz—PSG III), 1 January 2017	Implementation of the agreed recommendations developed in a Federal-Länder working group on strengthening the role of the municipalities in long-term care between the Federal Government, the Länder and municipal umbrella organizations, introduced the new concept of the need for long-term care in social assistance law
Pflegepersonal-Stärkungsgesetz (PpSG), 1 January 2019	No upper limit for additional funding and elimination of the hospitals' own contribution, hospital reimbursement will be changed to a combination of flat rates per case and reimbursement of nursing staff costs from 2020, within the framework of the long-term care budget, the training allowances of trainees in pediatric nursing, nursing and nursing auxiliaries will be fully refinanced by the funding agencies in the first year of training from 2019

(*continued*)

Table 6.3 (continued)

Reform	Main reform content
Terminservice- und Versorgungsgesetz (TSVG), 11 May 2019	Expansion of the appointment service points as central contact points for patients and be available 24 hours a day, 7 days a week, increasing the minimum number of consultation hours offered by panel doctors, in underserved areas, the associations of SHI-accredited doctors must open their own practices or offer alternative care, extension of the scope of services of the statutory health insurance to include additional offers: The health insurance funds will be obliged to offer electronic patient files for their insured persons from 2021 at the latest
Digitale-Versorgung-Gesetz, 19 December 2019	Apps can be prescribed by doctors, facilitate access for manufacturers: After the app has been tested by the Federal Institute for Drugs and Medical Devices for safety, functionality, quality, data security and data protection, it will be provisionally reimbursed by the statutory health insurance for one year, extension of the Innovation Fund until 2024 with 200 million euro per year
Fairer-Kassenwettbewerb-Gesetz (GKV-FKG), 1 April 2020	Development of the morbidity-oriented risk structure compensation scheme by introducing a risk pool and a regional component and by extending the assessment of morbidity to more diagnoses

Source: Summaries of reforms are taken from the original legal documents and the overviews provided by Bandelow et al. (2019)

a return to parity financing of health insurance contributions was already agreed in the coalition agreement and implemented with the Act to Relieve the Burden on Insured Persons in SHI (GKV-Versichertenentlastungsgesetz; GKV-VEG). To counter the constant criticism of a "two-class system of medicine", which has recently been increasingly reflected in the question of how long patients have to wait for specialist appointments, the Appointment Service and Care Act (Terminstellenservice- und versorgungsgesetz; TSVG), established a uniform appointment service center for specialist appointments. In addition, office hours for physicians are being expanded.

In addition, there was a particular pressure from emerging challenges of the shortage of skilled workers (especially nursing staff), drug safety, and slow progress in digitalization. Jens Spahn responded to the challenges in care policy with an immediate care program that creates 13,000 additional positions in inpatient care for the elderly and ensures full refinancing of these positions in hospitals. In addition, it was decided to decouple the nursing staff costs from the DRGs. Both measures were adopted in the context of the Act to Strengthen the Nursing Staff (Pflegepersonalstärkungsgesetz; PpSG. With a view to a planned comprehensive reform of nursing care, the conclusion of collective agreements was envisaged. In the area of digitalization, the most prominent innovation is probably the possibility of making digital health applications reimbursable by including them in the health insurers' benefits catalogue. In addition, health care providers will be required to connect to the telematics infrastructure by a specified date. The Corona pandemic has also spurred some developments, such as the electronic certificate of incapacity for work and the e-prescription (Digital Care Act (Digitale-Versorgung-Gesetz; DVG)), which is also linked to the electronic patient record that must be offered to every patient by their health insurer from January 2021. In addition, the BMG taken over a majority stake in the gematik, the company responsible for the telematics infrastructure, which was previously led by actors of the self-governance.

Compared with previous health care reforms in Germany, there are few similarities. The RSA scheme and the free choice of sickness funds were generally considered a success. Nevertheless, as early as 2000 there were calls for continuous adjustment of this scheme, for example with the introduction of a regional and morbidity component (Busse, 2001, p. 176). Jens Spahn complied with these demands in the Fair Sickness Fund Competition Act (Fairer-Kassenwettbewerb-Gesetz; GKV-FKG) and even made rhetorical reference to Lahnstein (Rottschäfer, 2019), but earned criticism from sectoral actors (Litsch, 2019). Although the reforms are based on two special reports by the Scientific Advisory Council on the Further Development of the Risk Structure Compensation Scheme at the (now renamed) Federal Office for Social Security (Bundesamt für Soziale Sicherung, BAS) (Drösler et al., 2017, 2018), in which some members of the programmatic group were involved, members of the programmatic group in particular see the reform efforts around Jens Spahn as a "rhetorical relic" (Hermann & Graf, 2020) at best. Hermann (2020) concludes that the program of a solidarity-based competitive order is becoming increasingly unrecognizable under the grand coalition. With the appointment of new members of the SVR-G and the Scientific Advisory Council at the BAS and the dismissal of Jürgen Wasem and Eberhard Wille, Jens Spahn has even directly discharged members of the former programmatic group, which can also be seen as evidence of the decline of the programmatic group.

Looking at the reforms in detail, one could most readily assume that the substantive relationship between the individual measures was shaped by the ministers. Gröhe focused more on strengthening prevention and improvements in care policy. Spahn, on the other hand, announced digitalization as a central topic right at the beginning of his term in office. However, the setting of priorities by ministers alone contradicts the idea of the PAF and the premise of programmatic groups. The ministers acted as individuals and chose these topics as central to themselves. They did not act in groups and certainly not in programmatic groups. Certainly, ministerial policy was informed by the support of advisory groups, but even these did not function as programmatic groups because they had no biographical connections. The new leadership department under Spahn in the ministry could have been considered a new programmatic group under certain conditions. However, with the exception of State Secretary Thomas Steffen, there were no biographical connections to Spahn, and these were not based on biographical connections that would have had a content background (e.g., in committees or commissions). It was rather the partisan connection that paid off here.

From a content perspective, digitalization alone does not constitute a program. Thus, at least the reform communication coined by Jens Spahn contains neither a clear naming of problems that are to be solved by digitalization. Nor does it indicate, with reference to a clear uniform name of a program, which concrete measures can be derived to solve these problems. Nor does it state the goals of such a program. Thus, the call for more digitalization itself does not yet meet the criteria required of a policy program of a programmatic group. While a reform of integrated care is currently being discussed, former programmatic actors claim that the idea of cooperation and integration had failed (Brandhorst et al., 2017). The pandemic has provided new impetus and, among other things, raises the question of cooperation between the inpatient and outpatient sectors, even in sparsely populated regions. From this perspective, the distribution of vaccines is also driving regionalization efforts, which are also aimed at optimizing integrated care while taking regional characteristics into account.

Here, then, the Corona crisis offers a window for far-reaching reforms that are probably better explained from an MSF perspective than by looking at programmatic groups.

The discourse-analytical analysis of potential programmatic actors reveals a strong reorientation both in the programmatic debate and among the prominent personalities. As in France, media coverage of health policy declined to a similar extent, so no further discourse network is shown here either. The content was also about topics other than finance, solidarity, and competition. After the 2011 reforms, care policy and prevention came to the fore as major topics. Finally, under minister Hermann Gröhe, a redefinition of the concept of the need for care was undertaken, which Daniel Bahr had not yet succeeded in doing. During the election campaign for the 2013 general elections, the concepts of capitation fees and citizens' insurance were discussed again, but neither was seriously pushed through. Health policy at this time is characterized by an astonishing cross-party consensus in which there are no deep conflicts because of the absence of financial pressure. This is due in no small part to the consensual policy of health minister Hermann Gröhe, which largely differs from that of Jens Spahn, who is more prone to conflict and interested in his own career (Bandelow et al., 2020). The transition of the income-independent additional contribution to an income-based model was also largely uncontroversial.

Only after the historic election in 2017 and the failed coalition negotiations between CDU/CSU, FDP and the Greens is this lack of conflict resolved. The SPD is entering the renewed negotiations for a grand coalition with the demand for citizens' insurance. However, this does not become part of the coalition agreement; instead, the negotiating partners agree on an honorarium commission (BMG, 2018). The strong dominance of party-political figures and high-ranking politicians is also striking in the health policy debates between 2010 and 2020. All publicly prominent actors in the debate are health politicians (Karl Lauterbach, Ursula von der Leyen) or were or are health ministers (Daniel Bahr and Jens Spahn). The discourse is almost entirely unpopulated by actors from various key positions in the system, for example, from the ministerial bureaucracy, academia, or actors from self-governance. Health policy is thus apparently not the subject of a policy program of programmatic actors, but shaped by party-political debates that only play a real role in election campaigns. The centering of health policy around the person of Jens Spahn is one of the main differences from earlier reform periods. This is not to say that the respective ministers were not strong personalities or that there were no political conflicts over areas of health policy regulation, especially financing. However, reforms in the past were worked out much more in the shadows of the ministers. The media analysis also reveals some interesting statements against the backdrop of the theoretical perspective of policy feedback effects. Franz Knieps. as one of the former programmatic actors, states that it is necessary to design reforms in such a way that they provoke new reforms afterward (Bohsem, 2013). The reasoning behind this is that every reform has loopholes for actors to use the regulations in favor of their interests.

With regard to the biographical trajectories, and in contrast to the investigation period between 1990 and 2010, the individuals who have occupied the formal positions in the health care sector in the last ten years to date are neither biographically conspicuous nor linked by commissions or common experiences and career paths. Within the last few years, the relevant department in the health ministry has been filled by changing actors following the legacy of Franz Knieps, from Joachim Becker to Sonja Optendrenk, who recently took over as head of this department. When Jens Spahn took over the health ministry, he institutionally restructured the ministry's organization by establishing a management department in which he primarily placed people whom he trusted personally and with whom he had a biographical connection. While the strong role of shared biography generally fits the logic of programmatic action, the fact that this leadership division, far from being open to external actors of the health care system, resembled a "closed shop" of actors working predominantly to push the health minister in his own political ambitions, did not resemble the construction of an overarching vision for the health care sector. While the minister's agenda can be described as programmatic in that it followed a clear strategy of digitalization and patient-centered reforms, it was not linked to a programmatic group.

This becomes even clearer when looking at those in key positions who also do not share a biographical history. The new board members of the GKV-SV, Gernot Kiefer and Stefanie Stoff-Ahnis, come from different sickness funds and were not part of commissions or expert groups, in which they could have been involved in developing ideas for translation into policy programs. The current impartial chairman of the G-BA, Josef Hecken, does have a ministerial career behind him and was part of the preparatory group for the 2007 reform, apparently benefiting from the ideas he came up with himself. In his new position, however, he is no longer involved in any working groups, but is implementing measures instead of preparing them. This is another sign that the programmatic group is being dismantled.

Based on the observation that there is no evidence of programmatic actors in public discourse or at the level of formal positions in the health care system, no anchoring examples can be found in the analysis of professional actor biographies. Instead, the analyses show that there may very well be actors who have reached their positions through programmatic groups, such as in the case of the GKV-SV or Franz Knieps' many years as department head. Even Franz Knieps' successor in this position, Ulrich Orlowski, is seen in some eyes as his heir. In fact, however, given the diminished role of ministerial influence on major health care reforms (in part because such reforms did not exist in this form), a decline in programmatic action is becoming apparent. Although Ulrich Orlowski can still be seen as a programmatic actor to some extent, as he is also linked to other actors in the programmatic group through publications (Orlowski & Wasem, 2007) and close relationships (Interview G5), his activity in the reform process was clearly less visible and influential. Although some programmatic actors continued to hold important positions in the health care system, their influence diminished after the formation of the grand coalition in 2013. Hermann Gröhe was a rather weak, consensus-oriented health minister under whom no major policy change occurred (Bandelow et al., 2018). Jens Spahn uses the policy field for his own purposes and ambitions to reach higher positions. He has even dismissed some of the former programmatic actors in key positions in the health care sector (Klein, 2018).

REFERENCES

Allen, P., & Riemer Hommel, P. (2006). What Are 'Third Way' Governments Learning? Health Care Consumers and Quality in England and Germany. *Health Policy, 76*(2), 202–212.

Altenstetter, C., & Busse, R. (2005). Health Care Reform in Germany: Patchwork Change Within Established Governance Structures. *Journal of Health Politics, Policy and Law, 30*(1-2), 121–142.

Amelung, V., Eble, S., Hildebrandt, H., Knieps, F., Lägel, R., Ozegowski, S., ... Sjuts, R. (2017). *Innovationsfonds - Impulse für das deutsche Gesundheitssystem.* Medizinisch Wissenschaftliche Verlagsgesellschaft (MWV).

Arnold, M. (2000). Die Zukunft des Aktukrankenhauses. In M. Arnold, M. Litsch, & H. Schellschmidt (Eds.), *Krankenhaus-Report 2000. Schwerpunkt: Vergütungsreform mit DRGs* (pp. 3–12). Schattauer.

Bandelow, N. C., Eckert, F., Hornung, J., & Rüsenberg, R. (2020). Der Politikstil von Jens Spahn - Von Konsensorientierung zu Konfliktbereitschaft. *Gesundheits- und Sozialpolitik, 74*(1), 6–11.

Bandelow, N. C., Hartmann, A., & Hornung, J. (2018). Winter is Coming - But Not Yet. German Health Policy Under the Third Merkel Chancellorship. *German Politics, 28*(3), 444–461. https://doi.org/10.1080/0964400 8.2018.1512592

Bandelow, N. C., Hartmann, A., & Hornung, J. (2019). Selbstbeschränkte Gesundheitspolitik im Vorfeld neuer Punktuierungen. In R. Zohlnhöfer & T. Saalfeld (Eds.), *Zwischen Stillstand, Politikwandel und Krisenmanagement: Eine Bilanz der Regierung Merkel 2013-2017* (pp. 445–467). Springer Fachmedien Wiesbaden.

Bandelow, N. C., & Hornung, J. (2020). Policy Programme Cycles Through Old and New Programmatic Groups. *Journal of Public Policy, early view.* doi:https://doi.org/10.1017/S0143814X20000185

BAS, B. f. S. S. (2020). Wissenschaftlicher Beirat. Beiratsmitglieder im Berufungs zeitraum 2015 bis 2018. *https://www.bundesamtsozialsicherung.de/de/themen/risikostrukturausgleich/wissenschaftlicher-beirat/ehemalige-beiratsmitglieder/ (last retrieved from 12 December 2020).*

BKK DV, D. d. B. (2020). Der Vorstand. *https://www.bkk-dachverband.de/bkk-dv/struktur/vorstand (last retrieved from 7 December 2020).*

Blum, S., & Kuhlmann, J. (2016). Crisis? What Crisis? Restructuring the German Welfare System in Times of Unexpected Prosperity. In K. Schubert, P. D. Villota, & J. Kuhlmann (Eds.), *Challenges to European Welfare Systems* (pp. 133–158). Springer International Publishing.

BMG, B. f. G. (2018). Neues Vergütungssystem für ambulante Versorgung. Honorarkommission konstituiert sich im Bundesministerium für Gesundheit. *https://www.bundesgesundheitsministerium.de/ministerium/meldungen/2018/august/konstituierung-honorarkommission.html (last retrieved from 15 January 2020).*

Bode, I. (2010). Toward Disorganized Governance in Public Service Provision? The Case of German Sickness Funds. *International Journal of Public Administration, 33*(2), 61–72. https://doi.org/10.1080/0190069090 3188776

Bohsem, G. (2013). Die Gesundheitsflicker. *Süddeutsche Zeitung, 20 April 2013.*

Brandes, U., & Wagner, D. (2019). visone. visual social networks. *http://visone.ethz.ch.*

Brandhorst, A., Hildebrandt, H., & Luthe, E.-W. (Eds.). (2017). *Kooperation und Integration – das unvollendete Projekt des Gesundheitssystems.* Springer VS.

Braun, T., Rau, F., & Tuschen, K. H. (2008). Krankenhausvergütung - Ende der Konvergenzphase. In J. Klauber, B.-P. Robra, & H. Schellschmidt (Eds.), *Krankenhaus-Report 2007* (pp. 3–22). Schattauer GmbH.

Brown, L. D., & Amelung, V. E. (1999). 'Manacled Competition': Market Reforms In German Health Care. *Health Affairs, 18*(3), 76–91. https://doi.org/10.1377/hlthaff.18.3.76

Buchner, F., Goepffarth, D., & Wasem, J. (2013). The New Risk Adjustment Formula in Germany: Implementation and First Experiences. *Health Policy, 109* (3), 253-262. doi:https://doi.org/https://doi.org/10.1016/j.healthpol.2012.12.001

Busse, R. (2001). Risk Structure Compensation in Germanys Statutory Health Insurance. *European Journal of Public Health, 11*(2), 174–177. https://doi.org/10.1093/eurpub/11.2.174

Busse, R., & Schwartz, F. W. (1997). Financing Reforms in the German Hospital Sector: From Full Cost Cover Principle to Prospective Case Fees. *Medical Care, 35*(10), OS40–OS49. Retrieved from www.jstor.org/stable/3767246

Cassel, D., Ebsen, I., Greß, S., Jacobs, K., Schulze, S., & Wasem, J. (2008). Vertragswettbewerb in der GKV. Möglichkeiten und Grenzen vor und nach der Gesundheitsreform der Großen Koalition. *Wissenschaftliches Institut der AOK, https://www.wido.de/fileadmin/Dateien/Dokumente/Publikationen_Produkte/WIdO-Reihe/wido_reihe_vertragswettbewerb_gkv_2008.pdf (last retrieved from 6 December 2020).*

Cassel, D., Jacobs, K., Vauth, C., & Zerth, J. (2014). *Solidarische Wettbewerbsordnung. Genese, Umsetzung und Perspektiven einer Konzeption zur wettbewerblichen Gestaltung der Gesetzlichen Krankenversicherung.* medhochzwei Verlag GmbH.

Cassel, D., Knappe, E., & Oberender, P. (1997). Für Marktsteuerung, gegen Dirigismus im Gesundheitswesen. *Wirtschaftsdienst, 77*(1), 29–36.

Cheng, T.-M., & Reinhardt, U. E. (2008). Shepherding Major Health System Reforms: A Conversation With German Health Minister Ulla Schmidt. *Health Affairs, 27*(Suppl. 1), w204–w213. https://doi.org/10.1377/hlthaff.27.3.w204

Deutscher Bundestag. (1990). *Strukturreform der gesetzlichen Krankenversicherung Endbericht der Enquete-Kommission des 11. Deutschen Bundestages "Strukturre form der Gesetzlichen Krankenversicherung".* Bonn: Dt. Bundestag Referat Öffentlichkeitsarbeit.

Deutscher Bundestag. (1999). Gesetzentwurf der Fraktionen SPD und Bündnis 90/Die Grünen. *Drucksache 14/1245 http://dipbt.bundestag.de/doc/btd/14/012/1401245.pdf (last retrieved from 23 October 2020).*

DGB, D. G. (2003). Mehr Wettbewerb in der gesetzlichen Krankenversicherung. Eckpunkte zur Gesundheitsreform nachbessern. *https://www.dgb.de/presse/++co++8df6db00-1559-11df-4ca9-00093d10fae2 (last retrieved from 21 December 2020).*

Dietz, U. (2008). Kurze Geschichte der Arzneimittel Rabattverträge und Mutmaßungen über die weitere Entwicklung. *Gesundheits- und Sozialpolitik, 62*(4), 41–47. https://doi.org/10.2307/26766849

Drösler, S., Garbe, E., Hasford, J., Schubert, I., Ulrich, V., van de Ven, W., ... Wille, E. (2017). *Sondergutachten zu den Wirkungen des morbiditätsorientierten Risikostrukturausgleichs*. Retrieved from Bonn.

Drösler, S., Garbe, E., Hasford, J., Schubert, I., Ulrich, V., van de Ven, W., ... Wille, E. (2018). *Gutachten zu den regionalen Verteilungswirkungen des morbiditätsorientierten Risikostrukturausgleichs*. Retrieved from Bonn.

Dyer, O. (2020). Covid-19: Trump Sought to Buy Vaccine Developer Exclusively for US, Say German Officials. *BMJ, 368*, m1100. https://doi.org/10.1136/bmj.m1100

Ewert, B. (2009). Economization and Marketization in the German Healthcare System: How Do Users Respond? *German Policy Studies, 5*(1), 21–44.

Gerlinger, T. (2010). Health Care Reform in Germany. *German Policy Studies, 6*(1), 107–142.

Gerlinger, T. (2014). Gesundheitsreform in Deutschland. In A. Manzei & R. Schmiede (Eds.), *20 Jahre Wettbewerb im Gesundheitswesen* (pp. 35–69). Springer Fachmedien Wiesbaden.

Götze, R. (2013). 20 Jahre Gesundheitsstrukturgesetz: Leistungen und Lücken beim Abbau historisch bedingter Beitragssatzunterschiede. *Zeitschrift für Sozialreform, 59*(4), 459–476. https://doi.org/10.1515/zsr-2013-0403

Götze, R. (2016). *Ende der Dualität? Krankenversicherungsreformen in Deutschland und den Niederlanden*. Campus Verlag GmbH.

Grimmeisen, S., & Wendt, C. (2010). Die Gesundheitspolitik der Großen Koalition. In S. Bukow & W. Seemann (Eds.), *Die Große Koalition: Regierung – Politik – Parteien 2005–2009* (pp. 159–172). VS Verlag für Sozialwissenschaften.

Hartmann, A. (2003). In T. Ostheim & R. Zohlnhöfer (Eds.), *Patientennah, leistungsstark, finanzbewusst? Die Gesundheitspolitik der rot-grünen Bundesregierung* (pp. 259–280). Das rot-grüne Projekt.

Hassenteufel, P. (2020). Handling the COVID-19 Crisis in France: Politicization and Policy Changes in a Centralized State-led Health System. *European Policy Analysis, 6*(2), 1.

Henschke, C., Sundmacher, L., & Busse, R. (2013). Structural Changes in the German Pharmaceutical Market: Price Setting Mechanisms Based on the Early Benefit Evaluation. *Health Policy, 109*(3), 263–269. https://doi.org/10.1016/j.healthpol.2012.12.005

Hermann, C. (1997). Wer steuert die Gesetzliche Krankenversicherung? Vom alten – korporatistischen GKV-Erfolgsmodell und der – neuen – "Vorfahrt für die Eigenverantwortung". *Arbeit und Sozialpolitik, 51*(7/8), 10–16. https://doi.org/10.2307/26889247

Hermann, C. (2020). Baseline gekappt oder: Selektivverträge im Nirvana der Beliebigkeit. *Observer Gesundheit* *https://observer-gesundheit.de/baseline-gekappt-oder-selektivvertraege-im-nirvana-der-beliebigkeit/ (last retrieved from 1 July 2020)*.

Hermann, C., & Graf, J. (2012). Die Verantwortung der Krankenkassen für Sicherstellung und Organisation der gesundheitlichen Versorgung. *Gesundheits- und Sozialpolitik, 66*(6), 27–33. https://doi.org/10.2307/26767216

Hermann, C., & Graf, J. (2020). Versorgungswettbewerb zwischen Krankenkassen – nur noch ein rhetorisches Relikt in der Großen Koalition? *G&S Gesundheits- und Sozialpolitik, 74*(1), 18–23. https://doi.org/10.5771/1611-5821-2020-1-18

Hornung, J., & Bandelow, N. C. (2020). The Programmatic Elite in German Health Policy: Collective Action and Sectoral History. *Public Policy and Administration, 35*(3), 247–265. https://doi.org/10.1177/09520 76718798887

Jacobs, K. (2009). Ordnungspolitische Defizite der Gesundheitspolitik. *Gesundheits- und Sozialpolitik, 63*(3/4), 26–31. https://doi.org/10.2307/26766915

Jacobs, K., & Rebscher, H. (2014). Meilensteine auf dem Weg zur Solidarischen Wettbewerbsordnung. In D. Cassel, K. Jacobs, C. Vauth, & J. Zerth (Eds.), *Solidarische Wettbewerbsordnung. Genese, Umsetzung und Perspektiven einer Konzeption zur wettbewerblichen Gestaltung der Gesetzlichen Krankenversicherung* (pp. 45–73). medhochzwei Verlag GmbH.

Jahn, R., Staudt, S., & Wasem, J. (2009). Verbesserung des Risikostrukturausgleichs als Instrument zur Sicherung der Balance zwischen Solidarität und Wettbewerb. In R. Böckmann (Ed.), *Gesundheitsversorgung zwischen Solidarität und Wettbewerb* (pp. 43–61). VS Verlag für Sozialwissenschaften.

Kamke, K. (1998). The German Health Care System and Health Care Reform. *Health Policy, 43*(2), 171–194. https://doi.org/10.1016/S0168-8510(97)00096-1

Kifmann, M. (2017). Competition Policy for Health Care Provision in Germany. *Health Policy, 121*(2), 119–125. https://doi.org/10.1016/j.healthpol.2016.11.014

Klein, L. (2018). Wille muss gehen – Spahn beruft neue Professoren. *Apotheke Adhoc* https://www.apotheke-adhoc.de/nachrichten/detail/politik/wille-muss-gehen-spahn-beruft-neue-professoren-sachverstaendigenrat/ *(last retrieved from 28 December 2020).*

Knieps, F. (2016). Gesundheitspolitik zwischen Wettbewerb, Selbstverwaltung und staatlicher Steuerung - Versuch einer Bilanz der Gesundheitsreformen seit 1989. In E. Wille (Ed.), *Entwicklung und Wandel in der Gesundheitspolitik. 20. Bad Orber Gespräche über kontroverse Themen im Gesundheitswesen* (pp. 25–36). Peter Lang GmbH - Internationaler Verlag der Wissenschaften.

Knieps, F. (2017). *Gesundheitspolitik: Akteure, Aufgaben, Lösungen.* MWV Medizinisch Wissenschaftliche Verlagsgesellschaft mbH & Company KG.

Kruse, S., & Kruse, U. (2006). Welche Rolle spielen die Kassen der gesetzlichen Krankenversicherung in der Gesundheitspolitik? *G&S Gesundheits- und*

Sozialpolitik, 60(11-12), 46–52. https://doi.org/10.5771/1611-5821-2006-11-12-46

Kuhlmann, E., Allsop, J., & Saks, M. (2009). Professional Governance and Public Control: A Comparison of Healthcare in the United Kingdom and Germany. *Current Sociology*, 57(4), 511–528. https://doi.org/10.1177/0011392109104352

Laschet, H. (2019). Vor 25 Jahren. Der Aids-Skandal und die Zerschlagung des BGA. *ÄrzteZeitung https://www.aerztezeitung.de/Politik/Der-Aids-Skandal-und-die-Zerschlagung-des-BGA-314223.html (last retrieved from 23 October 2020).*

Lisac, M., Blum, K., & Schlette, S. (2008). Changing Long-established Structures for More Competition and Stronger Coordination: Health Care Reform in Germany in the New Millennium. *Intereconomics*, 43(4), 184–189.

Lisac, M., Reimers, L., Henke, K.-D., & Schlette, S. (2010). Access and Choice – Competition under the Roof of Solidarity in German Health Care: an Analysis of Health Policy Reforms since 2004. *Health Economics, Policy and Law*, 5(1), 31–52. https://doi.org/10.1017/S1744133109990144

Litsch, M. (2019). Das ist machtpolitischer Zentralismus. *Gesundheit und Gesellschaft*, 2019 (3), https://www.gg-digital.de/2019/2003/vorstandsinterview/index.html (last retrieved from 2020 December 2020).

Manouguian, M., Greß, S., & Wasem, J. (2006). Die niederländische Krankenversicherungsreform – ein Vorbild für das deutsche GKV-WSG? *Gesundheits- und Sozialpolitik*, 60(11/12), 30–34. https://doi.org/10.2307/26766692

Manow, P. (1994). *Gesundheitspolitik im Einigungsprozeß (Vol. Bd. 16).* Campus Verlag.

Mätzke, M. (2010). The Organization of Health Policy Functions in the German Federal Government. *Social Policy & Administration*, 44(2), 120–141. https://doi.org/10.1111/j.1467-9515.2009.00704.x

Mehl, E., & Weiß, I. (2015). Selektivverträge am Beispiel der Hausarztmodelle. In C. Thielscher (Ed.), *Medizinökonomie 1: Das System der medizinischen Versorgung* (pp. 633–662). Springer Fachmedien Wiesbaden.

Milstein, R., & Schreyögg, J. (2020). Empirische Evidenz zu den Wirkungen der Einführung des G-DRG-Systems. In J. Klauber, M. Geraedts, J. Friedrich, J. Wasem, & A. Beivers (Eds.), *Krankenhaus-Report 2020: Finanzierung und Vergütung am Scheideweg* pp. 25-39. : Springer Berlin Heidelberg.

Orlowski, U., & Wasem, J. (2007). *Gesundheitsreform 2007 (GKV-WSG). Änderungen und Auswirkungen auf einen Blick.* C.F. Müller, Verlagsgruppe Hüthig Jehle Rehm GmbH.

Perschke-Hartmann, C. (1994). *Die doppelte Reform. Gesundheitspolitik von Blüm zu Seehofer.* Springer VS.

Rebscher, H. (2016). Die Idee der Solidarischen Wettbewerbsordnung - Ausgangspunkt und Entwicklung. In E. Wille (Ed.), *Entwicklung und Wandel in der Gesundheitspolitik. 20. Bad Orber Gespräche über kontroverse Themen im Gesundheitswesen* (pp. 47–65). Peter Lang GmbH - Internationaler Verlag der Wissenschaften.

Reiners, H. (1993). Das Gesundheitsstrukturgesetz 'Ein Hauch von Sozialgeschichte ?' Werkstattbericht über eine gesundheitspolitische Weichenstellung. *Jahrbuch für Kritische Medizin und Gesundheits wissenschaften, 20,* 1.

Reiners, H. (2009). Die Gesundheitspolitik nach dem GKV-WSG. Zur Dialektik von politischer Verantwortung und Wettbewerb. *Gesundheits- und Sozialpolitik, 63*(2), 11–16. https://doi.org/10.2307/26766897

Reiners, H. (2017a). *Die Reformfibel 2.0. Handbuch der Gesundheitsreformen bis Ende 2017.* KomPart Verlagsgesellschaft mbH & Co. KG.

Reiners, H. (2017b). Mythos Lahnstein. *Gesundheit und Gesellschaft, 20*(9), 23–28.

Rohrer, B. (2017). Von Rabattverträgen war keiner so richtig begeistert. *DAZ. online https://www.deutsche-apotheker-zeitung.de/news/artikel/2017/04/04/von-rabattvertraegen-war-keiner-so-richtig-begeistert (last retrieved from 15 November 2020).*

Rosenbrock, R. (1992). Politik der Prävention - Möglichkeiten und Hinderungsgründe. In R. Müller & M. F. Schuntermann (Eds.), *Sozialpolitik als Gestaltungsauftrag: zum Gedenken an Alfred Schmidt* (pp. 151–173). Bund-Verlag.

Rothgang, H., Schmid, A., & Wendt, C. (2010). The Self-Regulatory German Healthcare System Between Growing Competition and State Hierarchy. In H. Rothgang, M. Cacace, L. Frisina, S. Grimmeisen, A. Schmid, & C. Wendt (Eds.), *The State and Healthcare: Comparing OECD Countries* (pp. 119–179). Palgrave Macmillan UK.

Rottschäfer, T. (2019). Plan für ein Lahnstein 2.0. *Gesundheit und Gesellschaft, 2019*(3), https://www.gg-digital.de/2019/2003/plan-fuer-ein-lahnstein-2012-2010/index.html (last retrieved from 2020 December 2020).

Schillen, P., & Kaiser, C. (2018). Zwischen öffentlich-rechtlicher Aufgabenerfüllung und ärztlicher Interessenvertretung. In T. Spier & C. Strünck (Eds.), *Ärzteverbände und ihre Mitglieder: Zwischen Einfluss- und Mitgliederlogik* (pp. 125–150). Springer Fachmedien Wiesbaden.

Schwartz, F. W., & Mosebach, K. (2003). Gesundheitsreform 2003: Gesundheit spolitik zwischen Strukturreformen und Partikularinteressen. *Public Health Forum, 11*(3), 2–3. https://doi.org/10.1515/pubhef-2003-1984

Seehofer, H. (1996). *Unsere Strategie ist voll aufgegangen / Interviewer: H. Graupner & S. Lebert.* Süddeutsche Zeitung, 6 July 1996.

Seehofer, H., Dreßler, R., Henke, K.-D., & Cassel, D. (1996). Strukturelle Reformen im Gesundheitsbereich. *Wirtschaftsdienst, 76*(2), 59–71.

Simon, M. (2016). Zusatzbeitrag und Festschreibung des Arbeitgeberbeitrags in der Gesetzlichen Krankenversicherung. Entstehung, Entwicklung und gesundheitspolitische Bedeutung. *Gesundheits- und Sozialpolitik, 70*(3), 47–52. https://doi.org/10.2307/26766215

Steinkohl, S. (1999). Die moderne Mediziin - noch bezahlbar? *Süddeutsche Zeitung, 20 November 1999.*

Stock, S. A. K., Redaelli, M., & Lauterbach, K. W. (2007). Disease Management and Health Care Reforms in Germany—Does More Competition Lead to Less Solidarity? *Health Policy, 80*(1), 86–96. https://doi.org/10.1016/j.healthpol.2006.02.005

Sucker-Sket, K. (2006). Gesundheitsreform: Erste Zwischenergebnisse werden am 1. Mai beraten. *Deutsche Apothekerzeitung https://www.deutsche-apotheker-zeitung.de/daz-az/2006/daz-15-2006/uid-15711 (last retrieved from 20 December 2020).*

SVR, S. f. d. K. A. i. G. (1995). Gesundheitsversorgung und Krankenversicherung 2000. Mehr Ergebnisorientierung, mehr Qualität und mehr Wirtschaftlichkeit. Kurzfassung und Empfehlungen. *https://www.svr-gesundheit.de/fileadmin/user_upload/Gutachten/1995/kurzf95.pdf (last retrieved from 4 December 2020).*

Universität Duisburg-Essen. (2020). Lehrstuhlinhaber Prof. Dr. rer. pol. Jürgen Wasem. *https://www.mm.wiwi.uni-due.de/team/lehrstuhlinhaber/juergen-wasem/#vitae (last retrieved from 4 December 2020).*

Wasem, J. (1993). Der kassenartenübergreifende Risikostrukturausgleich: Chancen für eine neue Wettbewerbsordnung in der GKV. *Sozialer Fortschritt, 42*(2), 32–38. Retrieved from http://www.jstor.org/stable/24510321

Wasem, J. (2009). Wissenschaftliche Politikberatung und Gesundheitsreform 2007. In W. Schroeder & R. Paquet (Eds.), *Gesundheitsreform 2007. Nach der Reform ist vor der Reform* (pp. 247–255). VS Verlag für Sozialwissenschaften.

Wasem, J., Lux, G., Neusser, S., & Schillo, S. (2016). Berücksichtigung des Krankengelds im RSA. *Gesundheits- und Sozialpolitik, 70*(4/5), 15–20. https://doi.org/10.2307/26766226

Wenzelburger, G., Arndt, C., & Jensen, C. (2018). Sozialstaatliche Kürzungspolitik in Deutschland: Nur eine Mär? Eine quantitative Gesetzgebungsanalyse 1974–2014. *Politische Vierteljahresschrift, 59*(4), 681–712. https://doi.org/10.1007/s11615-018-0109-5

Wolfangel, E. (2020). Der Unermüdliche. *AOK Baden-Württemberg https://www.aok.de/kp/bw/unternehmensbericht/der-unermuedliche/ (last retrieved from 7 December 2020).*

Wysong, J. A., & Abel, T. (1996). Risk Equalization, Competition, and Choice: A Preliminary Assessment of the 1993 German Health Reforms. *Sozial- und Präventivmedizin, 41*(4), 212–223. https://doi.org/10.1007/BF01299481

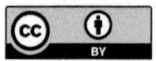

CHAPTER 7

The Institutions of Programmatic Action

What can we learn from these results of programmatic action analyses for the institutional conditions under which programmatic action generally occurs? To assess this conclusively in the case of French and German health policy, it is important to keep in mind that the theoretical perspective is born from the observation of French policy-making and is therefore initially strongly informed by the institutions of the French system. However, it is necessary to generalize the influence of institutions on the occurrence of programmatic action in order to enable traveling capacity of the PAF to other political systems. The institutions of policy advice and education turned out necessary in the interviews both with French and German experts. To this end, it is worth abstracting from specific national institutions. This is done in the following.

7.1 Institutionalized Elite Recruitment and Policy Advice—Par Excellence

Programmatic action in France is strongly influenced by the ENA, in line with the history of the PAF. The homogeneity of career paths and the biographical interfaces of programmatic actors are much more common in France. This is because career paths are more hierarchically organized and rigid than in other countries, including Germany. At this point, the elite formation system emerges as a key determinant of the formation of programmatic groups. In the health sector, moreover, the role of commissions, which are often established in advance of reforms, is confirmed in a special way. These expert commissions enable different but central actors in the policy process to participate in the elaboration of reforms and, in this way, to develop policy programs. The firmly institutionalized structures provide a quasi-permanent opportunity for programmatic groups to form. Here, a special role of the institution IGAS becomes apparent. As an institutionalized body of reflection, it is one of the first points of contact for the best ENA graduates. Not only do IGAS actors benefit from the institution's group-building dynamics, but they can also be appointed to other positions at any time from their IGAS position and then move back. This in itself allows for inter-institutional exchange and facilitates contact between actors who can form programmatic groups. At the same time, political institutions have hardly been subject to change since the Fifth Republic. Path dependency thus makes the formation of programmatic groups permanently possible.

Programmatic action in France is very executive-heavy and centralized because of the majoritarian democratic structures and few veto players. Programmatic groups are small and homogeneous, not only because of the elite formation system, but also because of the few points of contact between actors in the sector and at the subnational level. However, the empirical analysis here does not show that strong federalism and low corporatism must be obstacles to programmatic action. They may also enable programmatic action, because they involve fewer consensus constraints and allow programmatic actors to coordinate on a smaller scale. However, it can be concluded that the substance of the reform program makes less profound change possible as a result because fewer actors are involved.

With regard to the success of programmatic groups, which was the second focus of this study, the French political system offers fundamentally better opportunities for the long-term success of programmatic groups. Here again, the considerations on institutional influences on emerging and existing groups come into play. In France, hardly any distinction can be made between emerging and existing groups during the period under study, as they are recruited through established career paths and take the places of previous actors. The program thus becomes more institutionalized and emerging groups are the successors of the existing group, while the network remains the same. The political system, with its low degree of corporatism and federalism and few veto players, plays into the hands of programmatic groups.

Beginning with the selection of interviewees, 35 interview requests were sent to the actors identified in the chapters above. The selection was again guided by the formal positions these actors held over at least five years. Eleven interviews were conducted between November 2018 and May 2019. To preserve the anonymity granted, the names of the interviewees are not explicitly mentioned, but provided with an ID and the institution where they took place. Figure 7.1 displays the interview IDs and the respective institutions. Access to the transcripts of the interviews can be found in the appendix.

On the one hand, the interviews are suitable for cross-checking the previous findings about a policy program and a programmatic group that existed in French health policy between 1990 and 2010, and continued to have influence afterward. In terms of both the content and the actors of programmatic action, several interviewees confirm the interconnectedness. For example, a social adviser from this period in the prime minister's office notes:

> *F2: The reforms that have been carried out between 2007 and 2011 are really a continuation of 1995 and 2004. For me, they add, they change, but this is not a questioning of 1995 and 2007. Moreover, I don't have the feeling [...] that the Touraine reform finally really called into question this philosophy of the 1995–2004 years. (Interview F2, 2019)*

This is cross-validated by other interview statements.

> *F2: It seems to me that the two major structural reforms are the Juppé 1995/1996, and it is the 2004 law. So, we stay with that logic. The HPST law*

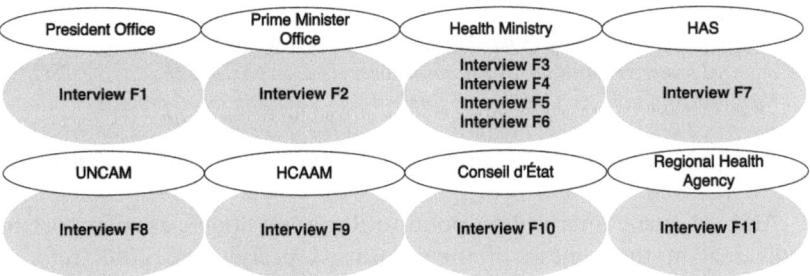

Fig. 7.1 Interview partners—French health policy. Source: Own illustration

is a change, but it does not call into question the policies followed since 1995 and 2004. (Interview F2, 2019)

Both statements reaffirm the great importance of the three reforms, the Plan Juppé in 1995, the Douste-Blazy reform in 2004, and the HPST in 2008. Beyond the reforms themselves, the interviews also reaffirmed the statements made as a result of the biographical analysis regarding the key role played by that several actors in the elaboration of these reforms. Specifically, the names that were dropped by the interviewees and that also appeared in the previous analysis of formal positions were Frédéric Van Roekeghem and Dominique Libault. As one of the project partners once stated: "[Libault] wrote > 99% of the Douste-Blazy law with his collaborator at the DSS" (Hassenteufel, private conversation). The fact that these actors, who biographically held key positions, were also decisive in the reforms that were passed justifies the positional approach, which states that actors in key positions play a dominant role in promoting policy programs. Moreover, the close collaboration between these actors leads them to develop a social identity based on their professional careers. Thus, the starting point for cooperation seems to be anchored in career intersections, which can develop into a programmatic identity if it is linked to a concretely identified reform program that is gradually adopted and implemented. This provides evidence for the biographical identity hypothesis.

F8: There was a trio on the implementation of the 2004 health insurance reform: Fréderic Van Roekeghem, Thomas and Jean-Marc Aubert. But on the HPST law, it was more with Olivier de Cadeville. It's on the institutional side, Dominique Libault. (Interview F8, 2019)

F5: Dominique Libault is the man in the organization of the ministry. It's someone who makes his whole career- (I1: Yes, in the DS.) in the DSS. (Interview F5, 2019)

F6: [Libault] tried very hard to launch reforms around both the universality of social protection and its sustainability over time, in particular with the CSG, the financing law, the CMU, and finally tried to rethink social protection in a universal dimension, but by maintaining, as [he] always sa[id], in the French model, an identity of Social Security in relation to the State. (Interview F6, 2019)

And yet, many interviewees point to Raymond Soubie as an important individual in the genesis of the reforms, especially the 2008 reform. Frédéric Van Roekeghem, "who knew music by heart, who was in Alain Juppé's cabinet in ninety-five, who was director of Mattei's cabinet in two thousand and four and who became general manager of the CNAM" (Interview F2, 2019), is associated with one of the major health care reforms, especially the 2004 reform, but also with the other two reforms. In particular, the influence on health policies that he exerted together with Raymond Soubie, whom he has known since that time, is also visible when other health policy actors are asked about this issue (see also Chastand, 2012):

> F10: *The Van Roekeghem-Soubie axis, in power relations, was nevertheless two goldsmiths. They are people who greatly influenced the policies that were made, there is no doubt about it.* (Interview F10, 2018)
> F6: *In fact in the immediate entourage then of Nicolas Sarkozy, President of the Republic, whether on health insurance or pensions, the one who really counted was Raymond Soubie.* (Interview F6, 2019)

The interview with a former staff member of Frédéric van Roekeghem also mentions other actors who were involved in the reform process. They state that collaboration with the finance ministry (Bercy), the health ministry (Matignon), and the presidency (Elysée) in preparing the reform was intense. They also explicitly name Éric Aubry as one of the key players in the health ministry.

> F8: *But very frequent with Bercy who was one of our allies anyway. [...] we were also in frequent interaction with Matignon and the Elysée. Matignon it must have been Eric AUBRY, at the Elysée, [...] Marguerite BERARD [...] Julien SAMSON.* (Interview F8, 2019)

Biographical connections become even more apparent here. While studying at the ENA, Éric Aubry was part of the 1980–1982 cohort that also included Anne-Marie Brocas, who participated in the Soubie Commission and later took a position in the DSS when the Plan Juppé was being prepared. This ensured that the policy program, once elaborated, lived on in the collaboration between the actors who formed a programmatic group around it and also placed several of them in key positions that were first established through this program.

With regard to the power resources that programmatic groups use for their success, the interviews reveal a particular relevance of certain institutions and networks. The results thus also confirm the relevance of the institutions identified as relevant at the outset, but focus even more narrowly on the CNAM and the DSS. One of the long-time members on the CNAM leadership assigns considerable power to the DSS in drafting legislation and assesses the CNAM as dependent on or at least subordinate to the control of the health ministry. It is often instrumentalized as a buffer against the interests of unions and health professions representative bodies, they said.

> *F8: When you are in the DSS, if there is a change in the regulations, you design the measure, write the text and monitor its financial impacts. [...] So, I would say that the CNAM's position was part of a somewhat complicated institutional and inter-ministerial game, but not at all beyond the control of the state. I would say that the role of the CNAM was rather to be in the front line, in a way also to protect the state on a number of subjects, particularly in negotiations with health professionals, which is a subject that can be quite costly.* (Interview F8, 2019)

The expectations that can also be confirmed is that a programmatic group uses the institutionalization of its policy program through institutions as a guarantee for the stability and survival of its ideas. Strengthening certain institutions through the policy program also allows them to place their members in the positions created by those policies. One interviewee in the DSS clearly states that the reforms have helped to strengthen the very department in which they were drafted:

> *F6: This whole '95–2007, 2008 phase is a very strong affirmation phase of the DSS. Well, I have to say—beyond the fact that I am a director in [*anonymized*]—I also play in this role. Now, quite honestly, I have a certain strength of conviction and this is a time when the DSS is very strong.* (Interview F6, 2019)

This interpretation is also cross-validated by another interviewee:

> *F7: In fact it allowed the Social Security Directorate, in a way, to become very autonomous from the decision in the health sector.* (Interview F7, 2019)

The interviews confirm, first, the results of the previous document analyses, discourse network analyses, and biographical analyses that the three major health policy reforms of 1995, 2004, and 2008 were interrelated both regarding the content and the actors surrounding the reforms. Moreover, the reforms can be consistently traced to multiple reports and working commissions in which the same actors prepared and subsequently pursued the jointly developed proposals that compose the policy program. Because the interviews highlighted the specific role of IGAS and DSS in the recruitment of career actors, they provide evidence for the biographical identity hypothesis and the science policy hypothesis. Consequently, these two institutions prove to be central to the careers of programmatic actors:

> F8: *I would say the world of social and the world of social budgets, it's a small world. So, most of the profiles went through IGAS or the DSS. So, the positions are held by people who have the same culture, the same profiles.* (Interview F8, 2019)

The career paths of policy actors, the institutions through which they pass, appear as a predisposition for the emergence of programmatic actors. In particular, some identified positions develop as turning points in the careers of individuals and as a central point in the education of individuals, which is the basis for the formation of programmatic groups.

> F5: *Well, the IGAS is a caricature of what the French technocratic system is like. They are people who do the ENA, they come out well ranked at the end of the ENA, and they will have the opportunity to have a golden parachute because they do a few years as inspectors. [...] They do this job for a few years, and then they take positions of responsibility in the Administration or in the operators who are around the Administration. And they come back—so it's a great thing because it means you can come in and out whenever you want.* (Interview F5, 2019)

In addition to the homogeneity of careers, which emerges here as a central factor for collaboration and ongoing careers, there is a need to bring these actors together for intellectual reflection and development of strategies. For such purposes, it is necessary to create bodies that institutionalize such efforts. Newly created institutions with many types of actors involved are one way to achieve this goal. Or, as one long-time DSS member states:

> F6: *The idea was to find bodies in which there is dialogue, consultation, information, cold reflection, and so these high councils, we started with the HCAAM in two thousand and four, or rather the COR first of all, excuse me, the COR, the HCAAM, the family council, the HCFiPS and I think it plays a useful role. I was also talking about the fact that administrations are often taken by urgency, that there is nevertheless a lack of strategic thinking that I find a little strong today in the system and the high councils can make it possible to bring a little strategic thinking with resources that are quite limited in the end, to pro-*

pose medium-term visions. For example, the HCAAM, the recent HCAAM report on the health system, nevertheless inspired the health law quite a bit. (Interview F6, 2019)

Besides, the question of where content of policy programs comes from is a key element in the analysis of programmatic action. In the previous chapter, the occurrence of programmatic action revealed the importance of working commissions in bringing together actors who later use the policy program to place themselves in the key power positions in which they implement that program. Key institutions where policy proposals are developed include IGAS and the directorates in the health ministry, DSS, (Direction de la Recherche, des Études, de l'Évaluation et des Statistiques (Research, Studies, Evaluation and Statistics Branch); DREES), and DGOS.

> *F5: There are many prospective reports because in fact it is much more used as a suggestion box [...] the Administration has been much strengthened in the study department since we created a studies department, the DREES, in the years two thousand, ninety-eight or ninety-nine, so there is a studies department at the Ministry of Social Affairs that also does evaluation, [...] and then there is a national health insurance fund that has study services. [...] in France the production of expertise and evaluation of public policy is done—(I1: At IGAS.) by the administration, that's it.—(I2: Internally.)—That's it.*
>
> *F5: What must also be said is that IGAS gives resources, expertise to those who leave it, which means that we are then very well equipped for political positions or responsibilities—*
>
> *F5: It gives you a general culture—that's it. [...] You know everyone because you spend your life meeting people in the field. (Interview F5, 2019)*

In addition to the well-known and established institutions, the creation of new institutions, including the HCAAM, during the implementation of the policy program also served the purpose of creating a new body for the generation of policy proposals.

> *F9: But in 2004, HCAAM was indeed created with the idea of creating a consultation process that allows proposals to emerge. (Interview F9, 2018)*

Besides the formally installed institutions, temporary working commissions, explicitly established for the preparation of health care reforms and composed of several actors who are repeatedly part of these commissions, play a central role in the continuous promotion and implementation of a policy program. Such working commissions, of which the Soubie

Commission can be considered the first, guaranteed the continuous participation of programmatic actors in the decision-making process and allowed them to translate their ideas into concrete policies.

F8: There was an actor at the time too, it was Gérard Larcher. Because Sarkozy had entrusted him with a mission for which I was the rapporteur. So I wrote Gérard Larcher's report after I left for the CNAM and Larcher even wanted to reunite the commission after when Roselyne Bachelot had drafted her bill. (Interview F8, 2019)

To conclude the French chapter at this point: The different methodological approaches, from the analysis of legal documents, media and public discourses, actor biographies, and finally qualitative interviews, cross-validate the findings on a programmatic group between 1990 and 2020. The reforms adopted during this period can clearly be traced back to a policy program and programmatic actors linked by biographical career trajectories and shared policy ideas. The institutions of programmatic action are located, at least in France, in central institutions of the education system, whose graduates have increasingly oriented themselves toward the top positions in health policy. Certainly, the French education system and the recruitment process of administrative and political staff through the ENA facilitate homogeneity of career trajectories and increase the likelihood that actors will eventually meet and collaborate. Such an education system is unique in comparative politics, but it explains how institutions can form the elites that later occupy key positions in the policy process (Hassenteufel & Le Galès, 2018, pp. 296-297). In health policy, the social security system has become a more prominent career path for these actors since the 1980s, as evidenced by the increasing number of actors occupying positions created in the health care system (Genieys, 2005).

In addition to the education system, the strong incorporation of advice and scientific thinking in the processes of decision-making can be observed in France. The bringing together of actors in bodies of intellectual reflection to develop reform proposals are ideal conditions for the formation of programmatic groups. This occurs primarily through the ministerial cabinets, which involve numerous advisors who can act as a group, but also through the IGAS, which symbolizes an institutionalization of the scientific advice fed into the policy process. Moreover, the institutions of ENA, IGAS, and the advisory and decision making positions in the ministry are closely intertwined, and actors frequently move between these positions.

In the study of French public administration, scholars argue that the resulting professional bureaucracies are characterized by great expertise and networking and a consequential influence on policy-making (Bezes, 2016, p. 260). It remains to be evaluated, against the backdrop of the German case, to what extent these institutions can be generalized independently of the institutions setting and the political system.

With regard to the long-term success of the programmatic group in France, one can conclude that the programmatic actors succeeded in networking in such a way that it was possible to consistently fill positions, even against the backdrop of political changes. The bureaucratic network is thus stable and independent of macropolitical changes, maintaining itself through the very institutions that led to its formation. Indeed, this is due in large part to the educational system that predetermines these career paths. However, the programmatic group has also managed to establish institutions and new agencies (HCAAM, HAS) from which its members continue to benefit because they give them influence in policy processes and create positions that strengthen the network as a whole. Here, too, it remains to be evaluated for the German case whether such mechanisms exist analogously in other systems.

7.2   Federalism, Corporatism, and Institutional Change in Germany

In contrast to France, programmatic action in German health policy did not persist. This was due to institutional changes, but also due to particular institutional settings and lacking institutions of elite building and policy advice as the following paragraphs will show.

Federalism reforms have weakened the requirement for consent and thus the need to involve subnational actors in health policy decisions (Zohlnhöfer, 2009, p. 58). In German health policy, only reforms that affect the organization of hospital policy require approval by the Bundesrat (Bandelow et al., 2020). Even in the early stages of programmatic action, Rudolf Dreßler announced in 1996 that he would appeal to the mediation committee for the reforms planned by the black-yellow coalition, threatening to instrumentalize federalist structures. Nevertheless, the subnational level is not to be neglected, as it most recently represented a countervailing power again in the discussion about the supervision of health insurance funds. The decentralized structures in Germany therefore enable and hinder programmatic action in equal measure, as they promote group formation but tend to make success more difficult.

The corporatist bodies were also changed in the course of programmatic action. Institutions originally conceived as "bargaining corporatism" became "competitive corporatism" (Rhodes, 2001, p. 177), changing the traditional role of corporatism. Instead of negotiating social pacts, corporatist actors now compete more with each other and make decisions in the shadow of hierarchy, with the state playing an increasing role in negotiations. Parapublic institutions, described as another "node" besides parties and federalism (Katzenstein, 1987, pp. 4, 35), have been partially deprived of their role. Because of these nodes of parties, federalism, and parapublic institutions, the German political system offers several points of contact for programmatic actors. However, the formation of programmatic groups does not take place within these nodes, but rather when the nodes spill over and come together in new institutional forums.

Moreover, the increasing importance of coalition negotiations for German politics also has an impact on policy processes. For example, most reforms adopted in Germany in the past were strongly influenced by the coalition agreement. In contrast to the expert commissions that were very common in the past, the access of non-political actors to the elaboration of policy ideas is currently often realized through coalition negotiations—if they manage to enter them.

Findings from the previous analyses suggest that programmatic action occurred during the first period under study (1990–2010), but not in the second period under study (2011–2020), unlike in France. A qualitative analysis through interviews is intended to confirm these findings for the German case and shed more light on the resources, strategies, and power of the programmatic group. To this end, a total of 37 interview inquiries were sent out and 20 Interviews were conducted between May 2018 and January 2020. Not all of these were conducted in the formally relevant institutions as shown in Fig. 7.2; some served as key informant interviews and some served to understand the underlying structure of the health care system. Figure 7.2 visualizes the interview IDs according to the institution to which the interviewee belongs. The remaining six interviews cannot clearly be assigned to one of the institutions. All are available from the appendix.

Federalism and corporatism were crucial to the success of the programmatic group. The role of the subnational states in this phase of programmatic action is relevant in that the arena of the Bundesrat and state

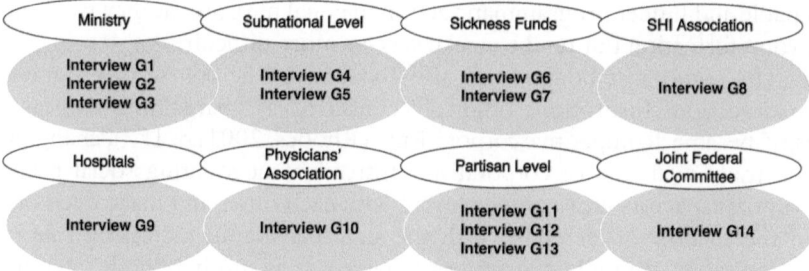

Fig. 7.2 Interview partners—German health policy. Source: Own illustration. The figure only shows the 14 interviews that have been conducted in key institutions of the health care system. The other six interview partners not included in this figure were experts from within the system that are, however, not clearly assigned to a particular institution

coordination was actively used to introduce the ideas of the Enquete Commission into the political process. The fact that the programmatic group occupied central positions in the states enabled it to coordinate as a group at that level as well, and to use the resources and decision-making processes at state level directly:

> *G6: And then we built up, as it were, a counter position, a reform perspective for the SHI system. And we fed that into the A-country process. And of course we made massive use of the findings of the Enquete. (Interview G6, 2019)*

Corporatism has an ambivalent role. On the one hand, the major reforms in the 1990s were deliberately adopted without the participation of stakeholders and the powerful actors from sickness funds and physicians' associations in order to directly overcome the expected resistance. On the other hand, the positive list, which was adopted and then not implemented, showed that the success of reforms adopted by political actors in retrospect depends on their implementation by self-governance. The interviews suggest that implementation is one of the biggest problems facing self-governance when it comes to health care reform. As a consequence, the analysis shows that in corporatist settings it is necessary for programmatic groups to involve corporatist actors who ensure broad support for the policy program. In doing so, they fulfill the original function of corporatist actors to communicate decisions to their members.

G1: And we then had a quasi-supervisory discussion with the GKV-SV and said: "So if you don't do it yourself, then we will have to do it ourselves in the near future or change the law". Then the other party said: "You know, you can change the law as often as you want. If we don't want to do it, we won't do it". (Interview G1, 2020)

At the same time, however, the German health care system is so centrally and closely organized that the respective actors, in constant exchange with each other, are quite capable of jointly implementing reforms with a common goal, as long as the corresponding interests are largely safeguarded. However, these exchanges are becoming increasingly informal and rarely allow for far-reaching reforms. Instead, these encounters can be described as everyday business.

G3: Let me say that we are dealing with a centrally managed health care system. So it's like the GDR (German Democratic Republic): small, healthy, yes? And that simply means that the staff of the ministry and the staff of the self-government know each other. [...] So in the informal sector, it is incredibly tight. (Interview G3, 2020)

Bringing together the findings from the empirical analyses of French and German programmatic action in health policy thus makes it possible to show which institutions are similar in the two otherwise highly different countries and could thus be generalizable as institutional conditions that favor or hinder programmatic action. However, in order to conclusively assess which institutions enable or block programmatic action, it is also necessary to provide a case in which the PAF is refuted and programmatic action did not occur. To confirm the institutional argument, one should then find that the institutions relevant to the occurrence of programmatic action are not present in the case under study. Therefore, the following subchapter uses expert interviews to ask about the reasons for the absence of programmatic action in German health policy since 2011.

The absence of programmatic action is also perceived by the key actors in the health care system and attributed to various factors. As much as the country level was used in the phase of programmatic action between 1990 and 2010 to feed policy proposals and the ideas of the Enquete Commission into the policy process, the states can act as a barrier. In the current phase, for example, there is a central need for reform with regard to cross-sectoral care and the question of how many hospitals are needed in which functions and at which locations. At this point, then, it becomes clear that the states can serve as both drivers and barriers to programmatic action, depending on whether programmatic actors are also directly at home in the respective structures:

> *G3: Unfortunately, I have to say that this is very much due to the steering of the Bund-Länder working group. If we don't have the solutions that we have, I don't think we can get them in the first few months. There's a real gap because you can only do this with the states, because we have to get to the hospitals and that's why you can't do it alone, so there has to be an agreement with the states.* (Interview G3, 2020)
>
> *G4: Many things really did work better at state level in the past. We were better organized, [...]. The Conference of Health Ministers simply signed off, in my view. [...] And this is, in other words, at their expense, although on the other hand, the real problems we have cannot be solved without the participation of the states.* (Interview G4, 2019)

Stakeholders also report a deterioration in the relationship between the ministry and the self-governance. This is mainly due to the fact that, in the eyes of the current health minister, self-governance no longer fulfills essential tasks or does so inadequately. Obvious examples are the lack of progress in the area of digitalization, which is criticized, but also the mutual blockades and hostility on essential questions of reimbursement and service provision.

> *I2: "Has the relationship between the BMG and self-governance changed in recent years?"—G1: "Yes, yes, deteriorated. That is the question of how to look at it. You can also say that it has improved. (Laughs.) No, the relationship is. So Spahn's statement in the committee: "I am in favor of self-government if it works."—I1: "So in this respect it [the state] has gained more control over self-government now the leadership than before?" —G1: "Yes, of course, it allows less and intervenes more often. The house finds this a bit ambivalent, of course, because it means more work. But in principle, we all think it's good not to be fooled. I think that is already the prevailing opinion."* (Interview G1, 2020)

A particular role is played here above all by the distinction between the scientific, factual, and subject-related level on the one hand and the party-political level, which is also partly state-controlled and oriented to the interests of self-governance, on the other. Several interviewees point out that the scientific level is responsible for the impulses, but these must then be renegotiated at the interest level. This is perhaps the biggest difference from programmatic action in France, which has to contend with fewer federal and sectoral interests due to its leaner institutional structure. These institutions were overcome by the old programmatic group.

G3: So there is always the phase where a high level of expertise is involved. Where one really tries to name and solve the problems and discuss possible solutions. And then there is always a second phase where the interests of the countries play a major role, which are very different. In other words, in terms of size, city-state countries, and so on. Quite a few things. Hospital structures that are completely different in Bavaria than in Saxony or something like that. And even if there is the CSU in Bavaria and the CDU in Saxony, there must be some kind of agreement between the two. And then the A- and B-states sit among themselves and try to agree on a line based on the professionalism of the work and then there is a question of colors and political exchange. And then the professionalism is moved back to the second row. Because of the compromises that have already been found. (Interview G3, 2020)

As important as scientific input and the involvement of scientific actors in reform processes is for the formation of programmatic groups and programs, it is dangerous if these scientific actors subsequently outlive their positions. It is true that it is of great importance for a programmatic group to create positions for its members. However, if these positions are not exchanged and become institutionalized over time, this is both an indicator of a programmatic group's success and a barrier to new programmatic actors seeking access to the system. In this respect, programmatic action thrives on ever new scientific impulses that must be constantly renewed and exchanged, just as science thrives on doubt.

G3: And there in the first place Wasem and Rothgang, who really did it to perfection. What I cannot blame them for. I begrudge them every cent they have. The problem is that they are becoming more systemic, have become systemic. Because the large number of expert opinions means that they have a pool of information that is no longer available to anyone else who is to work in the same field. And I think that is terrible from a scientific theory point of view. So that is... That is not possible. (Interview G3, 2020)

The current institutional conditions in Germany also make programmatic action difficult, as the institutional circumstances have changed considerably. The increased importance of coalition negotiations plays a central role in this context. The coalition agreements of 2013 and 2017/2018 are each characterized by a level of detail that offered the future health ministers only little room for maneuver. Hermann Gröhe, for example, worked out the measures set out in the coalition agreement in great detail. Jens Spahn does the same, but manages more than Gröhe to be known and visible to the public and to give the policies his own touch. The challenge posed by the Corona pandemic offers Jens Spahn an additional opportunity to present himself in public and recommend himself for higher office.

> *G5: But the last two coalition agreements were exceptional in the health care sector. They were so determined and so specific and so to the point, that is what we want. In the expression. In the form. Up to that point. There was not before in any coalition agreement of the last decades. So. And due to these specifications—and then there is the fact that there were two ministers of health. Gröhe, who really worked through the coalition agreement to perfection. And also Spahn, who, in addition to his own accents, Chapeau, has finally worked through the coalition agreement one to one.* (Interview G5, 2020)

In the coalition negotiations themselves, there are also opportunities for administrative actors to exert their own influence on policy formulation. While this is limited at the subordinate working group level, this influence can be very substantial and its success often depends on the personal relationships of trust between the individual actors at this level. If actors at this level have a shared history or bond based on analogies, this increases their mutual trust and they are able to leverage their past cooperation—and possibly the ideas that emerged from that collaboration—to achieve major policy changes. Thus, the institutional shift in Germany toward coalition negotiations has also led to changes at the working level. Despite their similar design to the grand coalitionary compromises of the 1990s, coalition negotiations do not function as a group-forming and group-identity-creating institution. Rather, it is the case that administrative actors who have previously worked together can use coalition negotiations as a venue to push their proposals through—assuming that the politicians give them enough space to do so.

> *G5: How do we do that now with the health coalition negotiations? And the fact is that in such rounds, it is only the politicians who say that we have first, second, third - we have to have all that. And then they name headings and then they somehow say at a certain point, well, go ahead. And then [we] sat together in the evening and wrote down what they wanted. [...] Then we formulated what we wanted. And then we presented it to them. Then they said, yes, that's good. Let's go like this. So a lot of things are really on a level of trust.* (Interview G5, 2020)

Despite the prominent role of coalition negotiations for German politics, there are also repeatedly commissions in the health sector that are set up as a result of coalition agreements or that can also work out a reform informally, which is then implemented politically. Here, too, it is evident that cooperation in the commissions is essentially characterized by trust. Current examples of such commissions in the German health care system are the Scientific Commission for a Modern Remuneration System (Wissenschaftliche Kommission für ein modernes Vergütungswesen; KOMV) (BMG, 2020a; KOMV, 2019) and the Federal Government/ Länder Working Group on "Cross-Sectoral Care" (Bund-Länder-Arbeitsgruppe "Sektorenübergreifende Versorgung") (BMG, 2018; Fricke, 2019), but also the Concerted Action on Care (Konzertierte Aktion Pflege; KAP) (BMG, 2020b).

> G8: *Then there are more often commissions, even provided for by law, such as the Federal and State Commissions, which may not have a constitutional framework or anything like that and can legislate, but if they agree on a position, on a draft law, on key points, whatever, then that is how it will be.* (Interview G8, 2019)
> G5: *[…] and these are coalitions of people who trust each other, even if they have completely different political, let's say party books.* (Interview G5, 2020)

Knowing that these commissions still exist, one might question the statement that programmatic action is no longer present in German health policy today. De facto, however, the overview of health policy reforms, the discourse network, and the analysis of professional actor biographies suggest that there is no programmatic group that builds on common biographical trajectories and currently translates its shared ideas into policy. Instead, the powerful role of the current health minister and coalition agreements has been much more influential in determining health policy in recent years than social groups and policy programs. However, administrative actors can still influence policy.

> G1: *"Well it is clearly different, yes. In the sense that more impulses come from him. Which does not mean that you have less influence. The debate is simply broader, I would say. So, what I did not know until now was a minister who reads the central statements of the associations on the legislative projects all by himself and then tells the specialist level 'please do, please check' on each point. But that is what he does".* (Interview G1, 2020)

These findings lead to the argument that programmatic action only started in the phase between 1989 and 1992 and that the PAF provides a working explanation for policy change until 2011. Thus, German health policy can be explained using different approaches depending on the phase. Before the 1990s, there were no major reforms and health policy did not yet exist as a policy sector with a ministerial portfolio (Döhler & Manow, 1997). This was only achieved in the 1990s by the programmatic group, which then lost its influence in the 2010s. Since then, German health policy has been in a phase of pluralization and fragmentation of interests with little problem pressure. However, it remains to be seen whether the now pressing problems of digitalization and financing, accelerated by the Corona pandemic, will drive the formation of a new programmatic group. Currently, however, the scientific impulses that once enabled programmatic action are now stuck. Advisors work according to orders instead of their ideas emerging from free thinking. If such open-ended scientific exchange is not institutionalized, even the system's own experts will not be able to effect substantial policy change.

Overall, it appears that the PAF can be a working explanation for policy change, but it can also be refuted. Counter-evidence for programmatic action is the finding that the actors in a given policy sector act on the basis of preferences derived from core beliefs and that there is a normative (rather than programmatic) opposition. Empirically, this is sometimes clearly evident in the interviews: One actor said in the interview that he was closer to an actor from another party with whom he had worked trustfully for a long time, than to any of his party friends. If he had said that he trusts his party friends more, the PAF would be refuted and the statement would be more consistent with the ACF or partisan theory. Moreover, the absence of programmatic action can be shown by the decline of an existing programmatic group. If there is no programmatic group, the sector disintegrates into economic interests where there are hardly any biographical links between the acting actors and thus hardly any trust. The result is that the individual actors fight for their own profit within the rules of the system without developing a vision for sustainable reforms of the sector. If it had turned out in the current situation that Sonja Optendrenk, for example, is closely networked within the SPD and jointly develops programs in commissions with Lauterbach's research assistant, this would have been more indicative of programmatic action. However, these biographical links between central actors from different parties and interests are not currently to be found.

What has also changed in Germany is the institutional setting of coalition negotiations, which now play a greater role in shaping policy than was the case before 2013. In contrast to the French case, the programmatic group was not able to change the sectoral structures in the health care system in its favor, or if it was able to do so, it did not grant further recruits to fill the seats it had left. This is partly explained by the lack of institutionalization of the education system. In France, the ENA is designed to bring in actors who are already connected to those in power and educates them to fill those seats. In Germany, there are some opportunities for these actors to meet and establish similarly stable career networks. Nevertheless, this needs to happen more actively in Germany, for example in the context of unique opportunities such as Enquete commissions or working groups that also include expert advice, comparable to the professionalization of the French bureaucracy. Only then is it possible for programmatic action to take hold in Germany. If the programmatic group fails to create these opportunities, its success will end. And if these opportunities do not exist again, there is no new programmatic group.

While both the presence and absence of programmatic action can be observed in German health policy, the interviews conducted with programmatic actors and experts suggest the ways in which political institutions influence these phenomena. First, the extent to which a policy sector has not yet been touched by scientific knowledge may facilitate the generation and dissemination of new ideas to shape the system. Such an endeavor requires that the actors who interact have an equal starting position. The fact that the health care system in Germany was just emerging and evolving at the beginning of the 1990s, and the experience with failed reforms in the years before, were extremely favorable for the formation of programmatic groups. Nevertheless, programmatic action did not arise automatically here, but rather as a result of systematic involvement of scientific insights:

> G4: *that in the 1990s and 2000s we were such an unrepeatable network of health professionals. What we had in common was that, as economists, social scientists, or lawyers, we were involuntary pioneers because the health care system, and especially the SHI system, was a "terra incognita" in the academic field until the 1980s. [...].* (Interview G4, 2019)

Second, and related to this, the increasing reliance on scientific research and findings in preparing reforms had a substantial impact on programmatic action in Germany. Again, several expert commissions were created in the early 1990s to provide space and opportunity for policy actors to discuss ideas and develop reform proposals. The involvement of scientists in these efforts ensured an outside perspective on problems and solutions that could be taken up by the actors in these commissions. Scientific advice was therefore strongly integrated into the creation of policy programs.

> *I: "[…] do you think that policy change is above all also triggered by just such scientific impulses? Do you think that this is what is actually needed again?"*
>
> *G6: "Yes, I am convinced of that, I can see that. So, in the background, it is certainly also the case with many—I think that politicians who are not completely pigheaded will always seek the advice of scientists".* (Interview G6, 2019)
>
> *G5: So since I was there, we have always discussed the topics of the Council of Experts with each other and worked them out and then partly decided ourselves, but it was always a relationship like that.* (Interview G3, 2020)

By interviewing representatives of these institutions, the empirical analysis also allows an assessment of the relevance of these institutions by looking at the relative influence they had in the reforms between 1990 and 2010. The first thing that can be confirmed is the importance of the Enquete Commission, which was already shown in the previous analysis of the reforms. Some of the above interviews indicated above were conducted with former members of the Enquete Commission. It is crucial to note how often the Enquete Commission and the Lahnstein compromise, in which many of the former members of the Enquete Commission participated, are repeatedly mentioned by health policy actors as a point of reference when explaining the adopted reforms:

> *G6: And we worked more or less on the side, more on longer-term or more structural things. There were so many hearings and so on. And that's why there wasn't really much where we had direct influence. But it paid off in the long run, especially in topics like what played a role in Lahnstein and so on. That's where we did a lot.* (Interview G6, 2019)

In order to introduce the ideas of the policy program, the programmatic group used the connections it had built up through the commissions in which it had prepared its policy program. Some of its members, such as Franz Knieps, who was head of the key department in the health ministry, took a central position in the decision-making process. They were also able to work with high-ranking politicians, such as the then health minister Ulla Schmidt, to push through the proposals. With regard to Ulla Schmidt, the importance of biographical connections is explicitly mentioned by one interviewee, who had even attended the same high school as her.

> G6: *Clearly in the background, of course, we also tried to exert political influence, and not least through Franz Knieps and others, that then- and Ulla Schmidt, whom I of course also know, she graduated from the same, three or four years before me at the same high school in Aachen, Reinhardt-Gymnasium.* (Interview G6, 2019)

Examining a little further which actors were members of the group and for what reason, it becomes clear again that biography is the determining factor for programmatic action. Depending on their professional background, each programmatic actor was characterized by a driving force that led them to engage in and shape programmatic action. For one type of programmatic actor, it was their health economics educational background that drove them in their efforts to introduce competition into the health care system. For others, it was rather the experience they had in the health care sector and/or their party-political streak that led them to embrace the program of competition. Either way, their involvement in commissions and their cooperation made them a group, and the policy program was what their combined preferences yielded.

> G2: *While some, so to speak, by training economists, socio-economists [...] saw it from a competitive point of view, that is, ideological aspects, rather to create such a competitive order between health insurance companies and to further develop and optimize it intertemporarily, others, now also from my social democratic side, were driven by the injustice of the existing system.* (Interview G2, 2019)

Despite these different drivers of action, there was a common strategy in promoting the content of the policy program. This strategy was to use science and scientific methods and results to inspire and legitimize the reform program, specifically that of evidence-based medicine, at a time when the affordability of health care was a real problem. So, the programmatic group took advantage of the situation that there was an urgent need for reform because of the problem pressure, and answered that problem with an evidence-based solution that at the same time helped them in communicating reform.

G5: There was a time when the competition order was established for this reason. Because, basically, the competitive order should be the counterpart of this, let's say, eminence-oriented medicine. Competition means data, means clarity, as a stringent DRG [...] In the next legislative procedures, the points were still picked out and worked through on the basis of the Enquete on structural reforms. [...] We were able to see that politicians only acted when the financial situation required it, that is where we are with the topic, and if any external influences, the pressure was too great that they had to act, but no longer with a proper guiding vision and the big competition topic, that is long gone. (Interview G5, 2020)

7.3   Intermediary Conclusion: Institutions of Programmatic Action

By recognizing the different institutions that exist in the two countries and the fact that programmatic action takes different forms depending on institutional conditions, the empirical analysis has uncovered institutions that are similar in both cases and can be seen as the central driving forces of programmatic action. However, these institutions are different from those normally studied by comparative politics and policy process research. In short, the institutions relevant to programmatic action are those that bring together and enable long-term cooperation among hybrid actors active in different institutional environments.

The test of the hypotheses formulated in the theoretical part shows that the institutions often considered in comparative politics can have an impact on programmatic action, but are not crucial for the existence of programmatic action. The programmatic group in France has succeeded in permanently strengthening and perpetuating its policy program through institutions. The recruitment of actors to fill these central positions (e.g., in the DSS or UNCAM) also occurs reliably through these networks. Germany has also managed to create new institutions. However, these do not fit into the original logic of the system, so they are not congruent with the prevailing institutional realities and have become alienated. Consequently, programmatic actors are no longer to be found here. As expected, decentralization and self-governance, as well as the strong role of parties in Germany compared to France, have an ambivalent effect here. They can promote programmatic action when they complement each other—as happened in Germany between 1990 and 2010—and serve as a power resource to push through policy programs. But they can also act as veto players and hinder programmatic action. In France, the traditional non-participation of corporatist actors has repeatedly led to strikes throughout the programmatic action phase, generating resistance to planned reforms. Programmatic groups in the French majoritarian democracy therefore also face hurdles in overcoming sectoral or subnational resistance.

Nevertheless, a stable elite formation system and the institutionalized integration of scientific expertise into the political decision-making process prove to be relevant institutions of programmatic action. When these institutions are stable, programmatic action is repeated. However, if these institutions change over time, this spells doom for programmatic groups if they cannot use the new institutional structure to their advantage. Figure 7.3 visualizes the institutions of programmatic action that were present in both French and German health policy and to which programmatic action can be traced.

In the case of the relevant institutions of the elite formation system and the constant integration of scientific expertise, it also becomes clear that it is primarily the individuals who become programmatic actors who are active in different arenas. They succeed in linking different arenas and, as a programmatic group, in exploiting the different resources inherent in this linkage. In this respect, they resemble boundary spanners who span multiple arenas rather than multiple issues (Brandenberger et al., 2020).

Regardless of institutions, the role of programmatic groups also shows that they are particularly successful when there is high problem pressure and a need for reform in a sector. In both France and Germany, the financing of

	France	Germany
decentralization	X	✓
self-governance	X	✓
scientific impulses and policy advice	✓	✓
systematic elite building	✓	✓
phenomenon: programmatic action	✓	✓

Fig. 7.3 Empirical evidence in support of hypotheses. Source: Own illustration. Favorable influence of political institutions on programmatic action

the health care system faced growing challenges in the early 1990s due to rising expenditure. These were addressed with different instruments. While in France the effects of the financial crisis and, more recently, the Corona crisis put the health care system under constant cost pressure, the policy program implemented in Germany largely averted the financial crisis. In Germany, the measures introduced in the pharmaceutical sector and low unemployment prevented the health care system from running into financial problems. In this case, therefore, the policy program virtually abolished itself, since it successfully solved the problems and there was subsequently no longer any problem pressure for further programmatic action.

It also striking, however, that in Germany and France the discourse and apportionment of blame differed. In Germany, it was primarily the ruling black-yellow coalition at the beginning of the 1990s that was blamed for the failure of cost containment, with the SPD leading the way. In France, there was more of a conflict between the central government in Paris and the sectoral or regional players. This is sometimes also due to the political system, so that different actors have to be brought together in programmatic groups depending on the country. In contrast to France, the role of party-political actors is stronger in Germany, and many sectoral and regional actors must also be involved. Thus, the success of a policy program depends in part on the support of other groups of actors (Sciarini et al., 2021).

References

Bandelow, N. C., Hornung, J., & Iskandar, L. Y. (2020). Krankenhausfinanzierung und -vergütung als politisches Handlungsfeld. In J. Klauber, M. Geraedts, J. Friedrich, J. Wasem, & A. Beivers (Eds.), *Krankenhaus-Report 2020: Finanzierung und Vergütung am Scheideweg* (pp. 299–313). Springer Berlin Heidelberg.

Bezes, P. (2016). Challenges to French Public Administration: Mapping the Vitality of its Knowledge Sources. In R. Elgie, E. Grossman, & A. G. Mazur (Eds.), *The Oxford Handbook of French Politics* (pp. 243–281). Oxford University Press.

BMG (Bundesministerium für Gesundheit) (2018). Mehr Zusammenarbeit und bessere Vernetzung im Gesundheitswesen - Bund-Länder-Arbeitsgruppe „Sektorenübergreifende Versorgung" nimmt Arbeit auf. *https://www.bundesgesundheitsministerium.de/presse/pressemitteilungen/2018/3-quartal/sektorenuebergreifende-versorgung.html (last retrieved from 24 February 2020)*.

BMG (Bundesministerium für Gesundheit) (2020a). Honorarkommission für ambulante ärztliche Vergütung legt Empfehlungen vor. *https://www.bundesgesundheitsministerium.de/bericht-komv.html (last retrieved from 20 February 2020)*.

BMG (Bundesministerium für Gesundheit) (2020b). Konzertierte Aktion Pflege. *https://www.bundesgesundheitsministerium.de/konzertierte-aktion-pflege.html (last retrieved from 20 December 2020).*

Brandenberger, L., Ingold, K., Fischer, M., Schläpfer, I., & Leifeld, P. (2020). Boundary Spanning Through Engagement of Policy Actors in Multiple Issues. *Policy Studies Journal, n/a*(n/a). doi:https://doi.org/10.1111/psj.12404

Chastand, J.-B. (2012). "Rocky", le "ministre bis" de la santé. *Le Monde https://www.lemonde.fr/sante/article/2012/10/08/rocky-le-ministre-bis-de-la-sante_1771640_1651302.html (last retrieved from 16 October 2020).*

Döhler, M., & Manow, P. (1997). *Strukturbildung von Politikfeldern: Das Beispiel bundesdeutscher Gesundheitspolitik seit den fünfziger Jahren.* Springer Fachmedien.

Fricke, A. (2019). Sektorenübergreifende Versorgung. Wissenschaftler zweifeln am Konzept der Bund-Länder-AG. *ÄrzteZeitung https://www.aerztezeitung. de/Politik/Wissenschaftler-zweifeln-am-Konzept-der-Bund-Laender-AG-255222.html (last retrieved from 23 January 2020).*

Genieys, W. (2005). La Constitution d'une Élite du Welfare dans la France des Années 1990. *Sociologie du Travail, 47*(2), 205–222.

Hassenteufel, P., & Le Galès, P. (2018). The Academic World of French Policy Studies: Training, Teaching and Researching. In C. Halpern, P. Hassenteufel, & P. Zittoun (Eds.), *Policy Analysis in France* (pp. 295–312). Policy Press.

Interview F2 (2019). Interview on 9 April 2019. *Paris, France (translated from French).*

Interview F5 (2019). Interview on 10 April 2019. *Paris, France (translated from French).*

Interview F6 (2019). Interview on 17 April 2019. *Paris, France (translated from French).*

Interview F7 (2019). Interview on 24 May 2019. *Paris, France (translated from French).*

Interview F8 (2019). Interview on 11 April 2019. *Paris, France (translated from French).*

Interview F9 (2018). Interview on 14 November 2018. *Paris, France (translated from French).*

Interview F10 (2018). Interview on 14 November 2018. *Paris, France (translated from French).*

Interview G1 (2020). Interview on 3 January 2020. *Berlin, Germany (translated from German).*

Interview G2 (2019). Interview on 3 December 2019. *Berlin, Germany (translated from German).*

Interview G3 (2020). Interview on 21 January 2020. *Berlin, Germany (translated from German).*

Interview G4 (2019). Interview on 9 May 2018. *Berlin, Germany (translated from German).*

Interview G5 (2020). Interview on 17 January 2020. *Hamburg, Germany (translated from German)*.

Interview G6 (2019). Interview on 12 June 2019. *Stuttgart, Germany (translated from German)*.

Interview G8 (2019). Interview on 9 January 2019. *Berlin, Germany (translated from German)*.

Katzenstein, P. J. (1987). *Policy and Politics in West Germany. The Growth of a Semisovereign State.* Temple University Press.

KOMV (2019). Empfehlungen für ein modernes Vergütungssystem in der ambulanten ärztlichen Versorgung. Retrieved from https://www.bundesgesundheitsministerium.de/fileadmin/Dateien/Downloads/K/KOMV/Bericht_der_Honorarkommission__KOMV_.pdf (last retrieved from 23 January 2020).

Rhodes, M. (2001). The Political Economy of Social Pacts: 'Competitive Corporatism' and European Welfare Reform. In P. Pierson (Ed.), *The New Politics of the Welfare State* (pp. 165–194). Oxford University Press.

Sciarini, P., Fischer, M., Gava, R., & Varone, F. (2021). The Influence of Co-sponsorship on MPs' Agenda-setting Success. *West European Politics, 44*(2), 327–353. https://doi.org/10.1080/01402382.2019.1697097

Zohlnhöfer, R. (2009). Der Politikverflechtungsfalle entwischt? Die Effekte der Föderalismusreform I auf die Gesetzgebung. *ZPol Zeitschrift für Politikwissenschaft, 19*(1), 39–76. https://doi.org/10.5771/1430-6387-2009-1-39

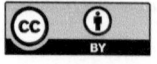

CHAPTER 8

Conclusion

The influence of institutions on programmatic action, and more specifically on the formation and success of programmatic groups, has been little explored. When studying the institutions of programmatic action, it is important to not neglect actors whose resources and interactions are moderated by the institutional settings, but who ultimately use existing resources—including law and legislative power—to achieve their policy goals (Radaelli et al., 2012, p. 547). Against the backdrop of the empirical analyses of the presence and absence of programmatic action in French and German health policy, this chapter summarizes the findings on the influence of institutions on programmatic action. What are the institutional opportunities and constraints for programmatic actors, and what are the institutions of programmatic action?

Drawing on the formulated hypotheses and the empirical case studies, the final question that remains to be answered is under which institutional conditions programmatic action occurs. Answering this question is essential for the application of the PAF in comparative public policy. The main argument that emerged during the study is that programmatic actors are sensitive to institutions, but that other institutions matter more than those known from the discipline of comparative politics. This does not mean that these well-known institutions do not also have an influence on the options for action of programmatic actors. However, the theoretical and empirical work has extrapolated two important institutional conditions

J. Hornung, *The Institutions of Programmatic Action*,
International Series on Public Policy,
https://doi.org/10.1007/978-3-031-05774-8_8

that influence the formation and success of programmatic groups. The first is referred to as socialization and elite formation, which is different in Germany than in France. Elites in Germany are socialized not as programmatic groups by definition, but as lawyers or party politicians. As a rule, they do not belong to a predefined group. Programmatic action is thus only possible if certain institutions allow the emergence of actors spanning several areas of the sector. The second requirement lies in the degree of institutionalized involvement of scientific advice in the policy process that stimulates the development of new ideas and policy programs. New ideas emerge from new ways of looking at the world, and scientific dialogue is one way to generate policy ideas. Therefore, the strategic and systematic integration of scientific advice in policy processes and decision-making structures is a key determinant of the emergence of programmatic groups and policy programs.

The analysis of programmatic action in France and Germany during the study period 1990–2020 has shown that programmatic groups occur under certain institutional conditions. France and Germany are institutionally very different. Consequently, the nature of programmatic groups also differs (Hassenteufel et al., 2010). In this context, programmatic groups in Germany and France may require different resources. In Germany, due to the strong role of the working parliament and in contrast to the rationalized parliamentarism in France, the realization of policy programs requires legislative competences and actors. Because of the different federal structure in Germany and France, programmatic groups in the former rely on the support of subnational actors. Also, the strong tradition of corporatism makes it necessary for programmatic groups in Germany to have actors and bodies of self-governance at their side, or at least to grow out of these systems. In France, programmatic groups are more hierarchical, centralized, and homogeneous, largely due to the system of elite formation and the centralized state.

In terms of content, it is striking that France and Germany faced similar challenges in health policy. Both countries were struggling with cost increases in health care system in the early 1990s, which raised fundamental questions about future financing and the services covered by insurance. Both countries also had the problem of excessively high drug prices, which could drive up prices without an additional benefit test, as well as overuse, underuse, and misuse with regard to the hospital landscape. As is well known, countries solved these problems differently, Germany by introducing competitive elements and an institutional restructuring of self-governance, and France by increased centralization and regulation, for example, through global budgets. It can be stated, however, that these crises of cost increase as problem pressure did not automatically lead to programmatic action, but certainly triggered it. In addition, health care reforms in both France and Germany have resulted in a stronger role for the state and a more hierarchical mode of governance to the detriment of self-governance (Bandelow, 2009).

Despite these differences, the analysis has brought to light generalizable institutions that function analogously in institutionally very different countries—such as Germany and France. While the design of these institutions determines the characteristics of programmatic groups, their existence can be demonstrated on a country-specific basis and the presumed influence on programmatic action remains. In accordance with the formulated hypotheses, the following influences of institutions on programmatic action can thus be concluded.

8.1   THE INSTITUTIONS OF PAF

The relevant institutions of the PAF were narrowed down to two main aspects, namely the recruitment processes and career paths of administrative actors and the institutionalization of expert advice in the policy process, which is related to the former. Thus, the PAF confirms what Hall (1983, pp. 46-47) calls the four institutional conditions conducive to policy innovation: centralization of power in a few hands, concentration of power in the executive branch (although Hall points out that political leaders rather than civil servants should be seen as initiators of innovation), access to information and expertise, and active collaboration through informal alliances between politicians and civil servants. The PAF adds value to policy process research by providing a theoretical lens that focuses its attention on precisely these processes that are relevant to major policy change.

In France, the process of elite formation is very formal. ENA institutions serve to train bureaucrats and politicians who will later significantly shape policy decisions and programs. In Germany, it was mainly informal networks that were formed through formal institutions (Enquete Commission), but then became more and more entrenched until they were no longer entrenched. This shows that in countries with formalized elite-forming structures and institutions that ensure group formation across political and interest-driven perspectives, that is, especially with reference to science, programmatic action is clearly more predictable and longer term. In countries where these structures do not exist, informal networks are more common and can form programmatic groups over the long term. However, these come to an end if they do not perpetuate their exchanges. The Enquete Commission in Germany is described by those involved as unique.

For the generation of policy programs and ideas, the involvement of scientific expertise proves to be a necessary condition for programmatic action. Innovative policy programs need impetus to enable the development of such programs. However, progressive and new ideas are almost exclusively due to new insights and perspectives that often emerge from dialogue and scientific advancement. In France, the integration of expertise into the political system, and especially into health policy, is much more institutionalized through the ministerial cabinets and the IGAS. In France, thus, this occurred through exchanges between members of ministerial cabinets, that is, the bureaucrats in the ministry with their close ties to other sectoral actors, to whom they are often still linked through the institution of the ENA (Gaffney, 1991, p. 9). In Germany, the Enquete Commission and other commissions following this expert body represent an artificially created institutionalization of expert advice and a point of biographical commonality that functioned analogously as a generator of programmatic action. The institutions of programmatic action may thus not be preexistent to begin with, but they can be—and empirical evidence shows that they are—created as a functional equivalent that triggers programmatic action. It is true that German also has long-term bodies for the integration of scientific findings in the form of the SVR-G and the Scientific Advisory Board for the Further Development of the Morbi-RSA at the BAS. However, these scientific institutions work directly on behalf of the BMG. "Free thinking", as is the case in France, is therefore hardly possible. This was created uniquely in Germany by the Enquete Commission. Furthermore, while these bodies in Germany are institutionalized, there are no institutionalized career paths leading directly to it. The programmatic group has thus also failed to use this institution for its interests in the long term.

8.2 Programmatic Action and Political Institutions of Power

A key question about the influence of political institutions on programmatic action concerned the ways in which *federal and subnational institutions* affect group formation and influence actors at different levels of policy-making. This question is also relevant from the perspective of veto players, as the Bundesrat is an institutional veto player in Germany. In this respect, France and Germany represented two different institutional settings, with Germany characterized by its distinct subnational structures of policy-making and France by its centralized majoritarian democracy. From the perspective of theoretical considerations, it was initially unclear whether federalist structures tend to favor or hinder the possibility of programmatic group formation. Empirical analysis has shown that both can be the case. Indeed, in states with a strong role for the subnational level of policy-making, programmatic groups can profit from actors at that level by expanding the scope of action and facilitating the implementation of the policy program. More actors in key positions mean more power resources to push for policies and use different venues to pass them. However, if actors at the subnational level are opposed to policy change or a programmatic group's program, they will probably succeed in blocking these reform attempts. This is consistent with research suggesting a strong role of collective identity formation at the territorial level at the interface between federalist institutions and public policy (Béland & Lecours, 2020). In contrast, this risk does not exist when decision-making structures are more centralized and involve fewer actors, as smaller groups of individuals are more likely to band together.

Not only the number of actors but also the occasions for group formation differ by the degree of federalism. Multilevel structures allow for the formation of cross-level working groups and commissions to jointly develop solutions to problems that affect all levels equally (Benz, 2017). It is not uncommon for major health care reforms to have been prepared through consensus discussions involving actors from these multilevel structures. This creates both opportunities and constraints for programmatic action in particular and for major policy change in general: If actors agree on key points and a common direction for reform, as is the case with programmatic groups, the chances are high that the changes decided upon will have a substantial effect on the structures of the policy sector and that far-reaching changes are possible. If there is no such agreement, it is much more difficult for actor groups (programmatic groups) to achieve major policy change because there are many blocking points (veto players) that can hinder their efforts.

Turning to the *corporatism* perspective, a similar ambivalent conclusion can be drawn: Although the programmatic group in German health policy weakened the sectoral actors, it was the existence of associations and their strong role in the self-governance of the sector that enabled the formation of programmatic actors in the first place. Indeed, it was the scientific institute of the local sickness funds that served as a cadre for the later successful members of the programmatic group. The programmatic actors who began their careers in this institution and then spread to key positions at the subnational level, in decision-making bodies of the self-governance, or in the ministry shared a biographical experience that would bind them over the period of programmatic action. In France, the relationship with corporatist actors was less tense, partly due to the lower degree of institutionalized involvement of these actors in decision-making processes. Health reforms in France were accompanied by persistent strong protests by sectoral actors—a well-known phenomenon in French politics. This may explain why the measures adopted in German health policy were more substantial (but not permanent), while the French reforms were more stable but less far-reaching. Similar to the structures of federalism, then, the structures of corporatism cannot be unanimously assessed as either conducive or obstructive to programmatic action. Whether they prove favorable or not depends on the constitution of the programmatic group and the inclusiveness of the policy program.

In general, the empirical analysis has revealed that the openness of a political system (e.g., through many points of contact such as decentralized structures, corporatist structures, and a large number of veto players) can also form constant points of contact for programmatic actors. The examples of France and Germany also show that in Germany's political system, which is more open in this respect, programmatic groups "change" more frequently. At the same time, however, there is a greater chance that there will be no programmatic groups, since many actors must also be involved in programmatic action. Insofar, established institutions as well have a substantial impact on whether programmatic groups form and are successful or not.

8.3   The Challenge of Institutional Change

Having identified the relevant institutions for programmatic action, it remains to be stated that this is also accompanied by a potential influence of the dynamics of institutional change. Because the empirical study looked at political institutions in a policy sector, institutional change can affect both the political system and the policy sector. Programmatic groups may benefit or be hindered by these institutional changes. It is therefore useful to distinguish between sectoral institutional changes, which are often induced by programmatic actors, and political institutional changes, which may challenge an existing programmatic group or provide incentives for a new group to form.

As a consequence, an important conclusion regarding the institutions of programmatic action is that of institutional change and stability. Distinguishing between political and sectoral institutional change, one can see that the latter can be favorable for programmatic groups, provided that they are able to shape sectoral institutions in a way that is advantageous to them. However, the changing nature of political institutions makes it more difficult for programmatic actors to predict the institutional setting in which they operate and which allowed them to become successful initially. The programmatic group in French health policy changed sectoral institutions and strengthened itself and its members. The programmatic group in German health policy also changed sectoral institutions and placed its members in these newly created positions. However, the German political system has undergone an institutional change in that coalition negotiations and the resulting agreements that shape policies in the coming legislative period play an increasingly important role. As a result, the institutional conditions for programmatic action have changed. Programmatic actors now need to have access to coalition negotiations in order to get the content of their policy programs into coalition agreements, or they need to push for the creation of bodies that can be agreed upon in order to use these bodies later to achieve policy changes. The institutional changes in Germany can be seen as a major explanation for the decline of the programmatic group (Hornung, 2021), along with the insufficient consideration and inclusion of expert advice in policy formulation, and the lack of opportunities for group formation in elite recruitment.

Sectoral institutional changes often occur when responsibilities are redistributed, agencies are created, abandoned, or merged, and when structural features of policy-making are rearranged to alter existing decision-making procedures. If organizations and agencies are understood as groups of actors that also shape social identities (Gioia et al., 2010), the premises on which an organization is built also manifest the preferences its members hold. An agency charged with evaluating the additional benefits of treatments based on medical evidence will not generally question the value of evidence-based medicine. The strengthening of parliamentary oversight of health spending in France has paradoxically strengthened the executive level of the state, in the form of the DSS in the ministry. Moreover, when agencies are created, the bureaucracy often continues to influence policy-making through existing networks (Gains, 2003, p. 75). As a result, agencies have a substantial influence on policy-making (Bach et al., 2012), and policy-makers have an ongoing influence on implementation—the two spheres are not as separate as they may first appear (Verschuere, 2009). Programmatic groups can thus intentionally shape institutions by creating agencies and new regulations with those agencies that ensure their long-term influence on policy-making. The institutional rules that dominate a policy sector may likewise be adapted by programmatic groups to serve their goals. Thus, sectoral institutional change is profitable and important for programmatic actors.

In contrast, political institutional change tends to be detrimental to programmatic groups. If they have used existing political structures to advance to top positions, programmatic actors often lack connections to other venues and processes that may become more important as a result of institutional change. A prominent example of such institutional change is the increasing importance of coalition negotiations for the policies of a legislative period (Klüver & Bäck, 2019; Romeijn, 2020). This strengthens the political versus the administrative level of governance and gives more weight to the advisors and professionals of the parties involved in the negotiations. The politicization of reforms and the modes of negotiation—but at the political rather than the sectoral level—are revived to some extent.

One idea of the PAF is that policy programs can bring about institutional changes that underpin the ideas of the policy program, thus generating policy feedback effects. However, there is also the possibility that policies will be dismantled (Jordan et al., 2013), which is close to the idea of the end of policy programs. In this context, a feedback effect of a policy program can also be the dismantling of the policy program if it has proven inadequate to address emerging challenges or if other actors try to dominate a sector's policy with their own ideas. The PAF also argues for viewing policies as irrevocably linked to the programmatic group, which can also explain the rise and fall of policy programs (Bandelow & Hornung, 2020).

8.4 Limitations and Research Agenda

While this contribution has expanded research on the PAF and policy processes to include the role of institutions in programmatic action, there remain limitations and opportunities for future research that need to be addressed. These primarily relate to the falsification of the PAF both theoretically and empirically, the methodological procedure that relates to this falsification, and other explanations for programmatic action that should be explored in the future.

The theoretical and empirical part of this book also discussed how the PAF can be refuted, or more explicitly, whether biographical linkages systematically lead actors to cooperate and promote a policy program aimed at policy change. What the network analyses of both the French and the German cases have shown is that programmatic actors not only have biographical entanglements among themselves, but are also themselves characterized by biographical diversity. Thus, there appears to be at least one additional factor necessary to become a programmatic actor, which is the availability of points of contact with the various domains of a policy sector, including the bureaucracy, academia, and politics, as well as self-governance, where appropriate.

Related to this is the puzzle why some members of commissions such as the Enquete Commission and some individuals who share biographical ties with others have not climbed the careers ladder or become part of the programmatic group, or that some who have not shared these experiences have. Why is this the case? Why are there people who theoretically could have been (or perhaps should have been) part of the programmatic group but are not, and vice versa. The empirical study provides some starting points for answering this puzzle that need to be explored further. The first is that some actors simply did not identify with the elaborated policy program. It may be that they had competing social identities that prevented them from identifying with the programmatic group, or that some characteristics of the programmatic group made it impossible for them to integrate it into their social identity. It could also be that the frequency of contact had an influence here, namely that the contact between these actors and the programmatic actors was not sufficient for them to build trust and join the programmatic group. In addition to the social psychological determinants, a psychological finding of the analysis conducted is that personality plays a role in becoming a programmatic actor. This has turned out to be an ancillary aspect of the studied role of institutions on programmatic actors and therefore has not been further explored in this book. However, it seems worthwhile to research more about the psychological determinants or personality traits that make actors become programmatic actors, as these appear to influence the likelihood of certain actors to participate in programmatic groups.

Following this puzzle, a limitation can be named regarding the theoretical perspective of the PAF in general. How can it be prevented that the evidence produced in the empirical analysis is not inherently anecdotal, considering that the theoretical perspective grew out of the French political system, which by definition is designed to produce networks of elites that know and cooperate with each other? The actively created Enquete Commission also had the goal of incorporating expertise and enabling innovation from the outset. To be sure, this is the case. Nevertheless, the PAF offers the possibility of finding analogous institutional conditions that systematically produce programmatic action. Normally, the variance in the French and German institutional systems should provide different conditions for major policy change to occur. Nevertheless, the PAF formulates mechanisms that link similar political institutions to similar modes of policy change that go beyond purely rational logics of policy-making. It considers institutions that foster ideational thinking and group formation. Even noting that there are existing institutions that differ from country to country, such as party systems, one can assess that they perform similar functions in generating ideas and recruiting personnel, although this alone does not produce programmatic action. To do this, parties must be viewed in the context of the PAF institutions: The goal of a policy program is always to strengthen the programmatic group in terms of careers (authority and resources). This also creates new institutions. The program itself is interchangeable, as are the problems it is supposed to address. For example, France and Germany both had the goal of making the health care system more efficient. Germany has tried to do this through competition and centralization, France through hierarchical control of spending and territorialization with centralized competences. These are also sometimes the result of party effects or corporatism, or institutionalist conditions. Ultimately, however, the goals of the two programmatic groups were the same: career, authority, resources.

One way to overcome the danger of anecdotal evidence is for the PAF to follow a systematic and rigorous research protocol that also allows for evidence that programmatic action did not occur, such as in German health policy between 2011 and 2020. In terms of the methodological procedure, the order in which the tasks of the research protocol are carried out can be adapted depending on the research question. For an application in policy research, it makes sense to start with the analysis of policies with a view to a possible underlying policy program. Subsequently, the actors surrounding the policy program and finally their biographies can be explored. For researchers interested in elite studies and why certain actors become influential in the policy process and under which conditions, it seems more useful to begin by analyzing formal actor positions and biographies before examining a potentially shared policy program around which they have coalesced.

Also, with regard to the methodological procedure, the empirical analysis supports network analysis as a suitable tool for visualizing and analyzing programmatic groups. However, a distinction must be made here: A discourse network analysis based on media reports in daily newspapers runs the risk of ignoring the specialized discourses. Moreover, the actors appearing there are often assigned to the legislative or executive political level, depending on whether it is a parliamentary or presidential system. Depending on the political orientation of the newspapers, which in both countries was center-left, it may also be that policy ideas and/or policy actors are presented and selected for reports based on ideological premises. While the cross-checking of the results with interviews and document data suggests that the media analysis had a high validity, a potential bias cannot be ruled out completely. A future analysis of other media sources with different political views would help to present further evidence for the research question, and stress as well as explain potential discrepancies. Also, scientific experts or civil servants of the state apparatus do not always make it into this discourse. Discourse network analyses therefore serve in every case to identify a potential policy program and can also provide clues to a programmatic group behind it. However, this is not the same as the visibility of programmatic actors in a discourse. In order to visualize the connections between programmatic actors, social network analysis proves to be profitable in modeling the connections between actors through commissions and occasions for collaboration.

In health policy, there are other arenas and occasions that bring actors together besides those mentioned in the empirical analysis. However, these do not always turn out to be programmatic or lead to the formation of programmatic groups. The structures of federalism and corporatism and their associated venues may also be evaluated differently in light of the PAF. Until now, they have often been viewed from the perspective of competences and the prevention of policy proposals, that is, subnational and corporatist actors are present here mainly in the role of veto players. However, the PAF allows for understanding these structures as breeding grounds for new policy programs and to perceive their role in the cross-arena elaboration of policy programs. To this end, the diversity of venues allows for the identification of actors who populate multiple arenas and serve as liaison points between these structures, increasing the resources of the programmatic group to which they belong.

In addition to health policy, programmatic groups are potentially found in other policy fields. Previous studies show programmatic groups in defense policy and higher education policy (Duque, 2021; Faure, 2020). The institutions identified in this study function analogously in these policy fields: In order to research and analyze programmatic actors, it is always necessary to get an overview of the relevant structures of elite formation and group formation. The occasions and predispositions for these processes will differ from policy field to policy field. Furthermore, the PAF needs to assess the extent to which scientific impulses drive new policy programs. Again, this will vary across policy fields. However, generalization allows for comparable applications of the PAF across countries and issues. This is strongly recommended for future research projects.

More specifically with respect to health policy developments in France and Germany, the COVID-19 crisis clearly represents a turning point in the study of programmatic action as well. Developments surrounding the pandemic make existing problems in the health care system more visible. While the programmatic group is still active in France, programmatic actors in Germany have lost influence but remain visible in the discourse, for example, in thesis papers (Schrappe, François-Kettner, Gruhl, Hart, et al., 2020a; Schrappe, François-Kettner, Gruhl, Knieps, et al., 2020b), with first author Matthias Schrappe also being a long-time member of the SVR-G. The need for local solutions has triggered a potential reorientation toward greater regionalization of health care in both France and

Germany, combined with a greater focus on public health and the design of service provision (Hassenteufel, 2020; Hildebrandt et al., 2020). It is possible that new programmatic groups will form and provide responses to such challenges. However, for programmatic action to be initiated, a look at the PAF institutions teaches that the opportunities for group formation and involvement of expertise are needed. The COVID-19 pandemic also holds potential even in countries where institutions for programmatic action are less formalized or hampered by strong political parties, but institutions must prove conducive or be created to enable major policy change. It remains to be seen and evaluated whether this will succeed.

To conclude this book with a reference to the beginning: The Chilean change in economic policy is challenged at the end of 2019 by demonstrations claiming that capitalism has failed. Every program has its end, just as the era of the group associated with it ends when the main actors disappear from the stage. But while people can die, ideas can live on and new programmatic actors can rise to substantially shape policy sectors if institutions allow them to.

REFERENCES

Bach, T., Niklasson, B., & Painter, M. (2012). The Role of Agencies in Policymaking. *Policy and Society, 31*(3), 183–193. https://doi.org/10.1016/j.polsoc.2012.07.001

Bandelow, N. C. (2009). Divergente Stärkung staatlicher Steuerung von Krankenversicherungssystemen: Deutschland und Frankreich im Vergleich. In B. Rehder (Ed.), *Interessenvermittlung in Politikfeldern* (pp. 175–190). VS Verlag für Sozialwissenschaften.

Bandelow, N. C., & Hornung, J. (2020). Policy Programme Cycles Through Old and New Programmatic Groups. *Journal of Public Policy, early view*. doi:https://doi.org/10.1017/S0143814X20000185

Béland, D., & Lecours, A. (2020). Ideas, Federalism and Policy Feedback: an Institutionalist Approach. *Territory, Politics, Governance, 1*, 1–17. https://doi.org/10.1080/21622671.2020.1837225

Benz, A. (2017). Patterns of Multilevel Parliamentary Relations. Varieties and Dynamics in the EU and Other Federations. *Journal of European Public Policy, 24*(4), 499–519. https://doi.org/10.1080/13501763.2016.1273371

Duque, J. F. (2021). Who Embodies the Evaluative State? Programmatic Elites in the Chilean and the Colombian Policies of Quality Assurance in Higher Education. *European Policy Analysis, 7*(1), 48–63.

Faure, S. (2020). Defeating the Austerians of the Warfare State. French Arms Policy Through the Lens of the Programmatic Action Framework. *European Policy Analysis, 6*(2), 96–119.

Gaffney, J. (1991). The Political Think-tanks in the UK and the Ministerial Cabinets in France. *West European Politics, 14*(1), 1–17. https://doi.org/10.1080/01402389108424829

Gains, F. (2003). Executive Agencies in Government: The Impact of Bureaucratic Networks on Policy Outcomes. *Journal of Public Policy, 23*(1), 55–79. Retrieved from http://www.jstor.org/stable/4007757

Gioia, D. A., Price, K. N., Hamilton, A. L., & Thomas, J. B. (2010). Forging an Identity: An Insider-outsider Study of Processes Involved in the Formation of Organizational Identity. *Administrative Science Quarterly, 55*(1), 1–46. https://doi.org/10.2189/asqu.2010.55.1.1

Hall, P. A. (1983). Policy Innovation and the Structure of the State: The Politics-Administration Nexus in France and Britain. *The ANNALS of the American Academy of Political and Social Science, 466*(1), 43–59. https://doi.org/10.1177/0002716283466001003

Hassenteufel, P. (2020). Die Corona-Krise in Frankreich: zu wenig oder zu viel Staat? *Observer Gesundheit https://observer-gesundheit.de/die-corona-krise-in-frankreich-zu-wenig-oder-zu-viel-staat/ (last retrieved from 21 December 2020).*

Hassenteufel, P., Smyrl, M., Genieys, W., & Moreno-Fuentes, F. J. (2010). Programmatic Actors and the Transformation of European Health Care States. *Journal of Health Politics, Policy and Law, 35*(4), 517–538. https://doi.org/10.1215/03616878-2010-015

Hildebrandt, H., Bahrs, O., Borchers, U., Glaeske, G., Griewing, B., Härter, M., ... Wild, D. (2020). Integrierte Versorgung als nachhaltige Regelversorgung auf regionaler Ebene. Vorschlag für eine Neuausrichtung des deutschen Gesundheitssystems. *https://optimedis.de/files/Aktuelles/2020/IV-als-Regelversorgung_Vollversion.pdf (last retrieved from 1 December 2020).*

Hornung, J. (2021). The (Mis)fit of Policy Programs to Political Institutions and Its Influence on Programmatic Action – How Crisis Has Differently Hit French and German Health Policy. *European Policy Analysis, 7*(1), 120–138. https://doi.org/10.1002/epa2.1108

Jordan, A., Bauer, M. W., & Green-Pedersen, C. (2013). Policy Dismantling. *Journal of European Public Policy, 20*(5), 795–805. https://doi.org/10.1080/13501763.2013.771092

Klüver, H., & Bäck, H. (2019). Coalition Agreements, Issue Attention, and Cabinet Governance. *Comparative Political Studies, 52*(13-14), 1995–2031. https://doi.org/10.1177/0010414019830726

Radaelli, C. M., Dente, B., & Dossi, S. (2012). Recasting Institutionalism: Institutional Analysis and Public Policy. *European Political Science, 11*(4), 537–550. https://doi.org/10.1057/eps.2012.1

Romeijn, J. (2020). Lobbying During Government Formations: Do Policy Advocates Attain Their Preferences in Coalition Agreements? *West European Politics, 1,* 1–24. https://doi.org/10.1080/01402382.2020.1755515

Schrappe, M., François-Kettner, H., Gruhl, M., Hart, D., Knieps, F., Manow, P., ... Glaeske, G. (2020a). Thesenpapier 6. Die Pandemie durch SARS-CoV-2/CoViD-19 - Zur Notwendigkeit eines Strategiewechsels. *https://www.ndr.de/nachrichten/hamburg/thesenpapier104.pdf (last retrieved from 21 December 2020).*

Schrappe, M., François-Kettner, H., Gruhl, M., Knieps, F., Pfaff, H., & Glaeske, G. (2020b). Thesenpapier 1.0 zur Pandemie durch SARS-CoV-2/Covid-19. Datenbasis verbessern - Prävention gezielt weiterentwickeln - Bürgerrechte wahren. *Monitor Versorgungsforschung, 13*(3), 53–63.

Verschuere, B. (2009). The Role of Public Agencies in the Policy Making Process: Rhetoric versus Reality. *Public Policy and Administration, 24*(1), 23–46. https://doi.org/10.1177/0952076708097907

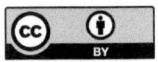